D1448213

**This book is to be returned on or before
the last date stamped below.**

15. MAR 1994
29 APR 1994

24 MAY 1994   1 2 JUN 2006   2 5 MAR 2018
                               - 8 JUN 2007   1 6 MAY 2018
22 JUN 1994
14 OCT 1994   2116/08
10 NOV 1994
                               2 3 MAR 2009
13 JAN 1995
13 JAN 1995   - 2 NOV 2010
-1 DEC
                               1 9 JUL 2011
10 JAN 1997
                               2 1 MAR 2012
                               3 0 APR 2012

VENABLES, G.S. et al.

Case presentations in
neurology

Other titles published

Case Presentations in Clinical Geriatric Medicine

Case Presentations in Endocrinology and Diabetes

Case Presentations in Gastrointestinal Disease

Case Presentations in General Surgery

Case Presentations in Heart Disease

Case Presentations in Paediatrics

Case Presentations in Renal Medicine

Case Presentations in Respiratory Medicine

Case Presentations in Urology

In preparation

Case Presentations in Anterial Surgery

Case Presentations in Heart Disease

Case Presentations in Medical Ophthalmology

Case Presentations in Otolaryngology

Case Presentations in Neurology

G. S. Venables, MRCP
Consultant and Honorary Clinical Lecturer in Neurology,
Royal Hallamshire Hospital, Sheffield

D. Bates, FRCP
Consultant and Senior Lecturer in Neurology,
Royal Victoria Infirmary, Newcastle upon Tyne

N. E. F. Cartlidge, FRCP
Consultant and Senior Lecturer in Neurology,
Royal Victoria Infirmary, Newcastle upon Tyne

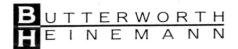

BUTTERWORTH
HEINEMANN

Butterworth-Heinemann Ltd
Linacre House, Jordan Hill, Oxford OX2 8DP

 PART OF REED INTERNATIONAL BOOKS

OXFORD   LONDON   BOSTON
MUNICH   NEW DELHI   SINGAPORE   SYDNEY
TOKYO   TORONTO   WELLINGTON

First published 1988
Reprinted 1991

© Butterworth-Heinemann 1988

British Library Cataloguing in Publication Data
Venables, G. S.
    Case presentations in neurology
    1. Man. Nervous system. Diseases – case studies
    I. Title   II. Bates, D. (David), 1942
    III. Cartlidge, N. E. F. (Niall Edward Foster)
    616.8'049

ISBN 0 7506 0444 1

Library of Congress Cataloguing in Publication Data
Venables, G. S.
    Case presentations in neurology/G. S. Venables, D. Bates,
    N. E. F. Cartlidge
    p.   cm.
    Includes bibliographies and index.
    ISBN 0 7506 0444 1
    1. Neurology – Case Studies – Problems, exercises, etc.
    I. Bates, D.   II. Cartlidge, N. E. F.   III. Title
    [DNLM: 1. Nervous System Diseases – case studies.
    2. Nervous System Diseases – examination questions.
    WL 18 B329c]
    RC359.B37   1988
    616.8 – dc19
    DNLM/DLC   88–5073

Printed and bound in Great Britain by
Redwood Press Limited, Melksham, Wiltshire

Preface

This book is intended for those doctors studying for higher professional qualifications such as the MRCP, although it may be of interest and use to medical students approaching their final examinations. Our intention has been to present a selection of case histories demonstrating how patients with often quite simple problems may present and to bring out aspects of their diagnosis and management. All the patients presented to the Department of Neurology including those with more obscure diagnoses. The book consists of 12 exercises each of six cases broadly corresponding to the style of the MRCP (UK) written case history papers and it is intended that each exercise should take about 45 minutes. Each case is set out with the history and physical findings given first. There follows either a series of questions or true/false statements on one side of the page which the reader should attempt before continuing on to the answer section on the other side. There then follows a short discussion about each case and a single reference. Neither the discussion nor the further reading is intended to be exhaustive and for further detail the reader should refer to any of the standard text books.

We would like to thank Dr K. Hall of the Neuroradiology Department, Newcastle General Hospital for the radiographs and Dr P. Fawcett, Consultant Neurophysiologist for copies of the neurophysiological investigations. We also wish to acknowledge and thank the Department of Medical Illustration and Audiovisual Aids of the University of Newcastle upon Tyne for the photographs, and thank Miss Fay Hannaby for secretarial assistance, and the staff of Butterworths for their patience in the production of this book.

G. S. Venables
D. Bates
N. E. F. Cartlidge

Abbreviations

ALS	Amyotrophic lateral sclerosis
BIH	Benign intracranial hypertension
CSF	Cerebrospinal fluid
CT	Computerized tomography
DVLC	Driver and Vehicle Licensing Centre
ECG	Electrocardiogram
EEG	Electroencephalogram
EMG	Electromyogram
ESR	Erythrocyte sedimentation rate
GP	General practitioner
γ-GT	γ-Glutamyltransferase
HSE	Herpes simplex encephalitis
ICP	Intracranial pressure
IgG	Immunoglobulin G
INH	Isonicotinic acid hydrazide (isoniazid)
MAO-B	Monoamine oxidase inhibitor type B
MCV	Mean corpuscular volume
NSAIDs	Non-steroidal anti-inflammatory drugs
PAS	*Para*-aminosalicylic acid
PTA	Post-traumatic amnesia
RBN	Retrobulbar neuritis
SSEP	Somatosensory evoked potential
SSPE	Subacute sclerosing panencephalitis
TGA	Transient global amnesia
TSH	Thyroid-stimulating hormone
VEP	Visual evoked potential

Exercise 1

Case 1.1 An impotent man

A 32-year-old man sought medical advice because of impotence. He had been married for 8 years and had two children aged 6 and 4 years. Previous sexual activity had been satisfactory. Two months before seeking advice he had developed total failure of erection and ejaculation, but claimed that sexual desire was undiminished. On direct questioning it was learnt that there were no morning erections and he had experienced frequency of micturition for 6 months and urgency for 2 months. On two or three occasions during the previous 6 months he had noticed a tendency to constipation. There was no past medical history, or family history of a similar complaint.

He was a healthy male with no abnormality on general examination including the genitalia. Neurological examination revealed normal tone and power in all four limbs but the tendon stretch reflexes were brisk. There were three beats of clonus at each ankle; the plantar responses were flexor.

Questions

1. What anatomical structures are involved?
2. What investigations are indicated?
3. What is the prognosis for improvement?
4. What treatment can be given?

2

Answers

1. Impotence commonly is of psychological origin. The combination of impotence with bladder and bowel dysfunction suggests an organic neurological cause. Anatomically, this may be attributable to a lesion in the parasympathetic nerve supply to the bladder, bowel and sexual organs, or secondary either to spinal cord or cauda equina disease or to an autonomic or generalized peripheral neuropathy. Certain drugs, e.g. methyldopa and β-blockers, can also cause impotence alone.
2. The neurological signs are non-localizing and not always of pathological significance. They exclude a peripheral neuropathy and, although it is unlikely that there will be structural disease involving the spinal canal, this should be excluded by myelography and the CSF examined for cells, protein and immunoglobulin content.
3. Impotence due to organic neurological disease has a poor prognosis and if it persists for more than a few months is likely to be permanent.
4. Mild sedatives and androgens have been used in treatment. A penile implant may assist in maintaining erections. There are encouraging reports of the use of implanted cauda equina nerve stimulators in producing both erections and ejaculation in impotent men. Ejaculation can also be achieved by electro-stimulation of the prostate.

Comment

Myelography was normal; there was a CSF pleocytosis with increased IgG, suggesting a diagnosis of demyelinating disease – a not infrequent cause of this combination of symptoms in young men.

Further reading

APPENZELLER, O., 'The reflex control of copulatory behaviour and neurogenic disorders of sexual function' *The Autonomic Nervous System* (1982). Elsevier Biomedical, Amsterdam, Chapter 16

Case 1.2 An evolving paraparesis

A 48-year-old woman presented with a short history of difficulty in walking and a tendency to trip over on the left leg. She had been unwell for 3 months during which time she had fallen twice, catching her toes on a kerbstone. There was no pain, but gradually her walking deteriorated and her friends noticed that she was unsteady. She had developed mild urgency and frequency of micturition. Two months previously she had, for the first time, experienced tingling in the fingers of the left hand.

She had seen her general practitioner at the age of 21 because of an episode of pain and visual impairment in the left eye, lasting 8 weeks; she had been told this was due to neuritis. There was no other past medical or family history.

General examination was normal. In the cranial nerves the only abnormality was left optic disc pallor. The upper limbs were normal. She had increased tone in the legs with a pyramidal distribution weakness on the left. Tendon stretch reflexes were brisk and there was sustained clonus at the left ankle. There was no sensory abnormality. She was mildly ataxic in both legs and on tandem walking. Examination of the spine was unremarkable.

Questions

1. These statements concerning this patient may be true or false:

   (a) Paraplegia following RBN is compatible with multiple sclerosis.
   (b) Her ataxia may be explained by a lesion in the spinal cord.
   (c) Delayed VEP and SSEP latencies would suggest multiple sclerosis.
   (d) Investigation should include examination of the CSF.
   (e) Treatment with steroids might be expected to reduce the severity of the symptoms.

4

Answers

1. (a) **True**
   (b) **True**
   (c) **True**
   (d) **True**
   (e) **True**

The combination of an evolving paraparesis and history of an episode of visual loss thought to be due to optic neuritis is highly suggestive of demyelinating disease, i.e. probable multiple sclerosis. The ataxia may be attributable to cerebellar lesions, but could also be due to disease in the cerebellar connections (spinocerebellar pathway) of the spinal cord. Investigations, including VEP and SSEP, confirmed disease at sites already established clinically and CSF examination failed to show evidence of inflammation or IgG synthesis within the neuraxis. Because diagnoses other than demyelinating disease may cause a similar spinal cord syndrome, further investigation to exclude cord compression should have been undertaken; however, on the assumption that the patient had demyelinating disease, it was justifiable to treat with corticosteroids as there is evidence that this may shorten the length of the relapse.

The VEP latency was delayed on the left. A delayed SSEP indicated a lesion in the cervical spinal cord. Spinal fluid opening pressure was 180 mm; no cells were seen; the total protein was 1.4 g/l of which 8% was IgG.

After treatment with corticosteroids, the patient's symptoms improved. At the age of 55 years her walking rapidly deteriorated and she developed pain in the fingers of the left hand. There was sensory loss to pinprick over the thumb and index finger of the left hand, extending to the lateral border of the forearm. There was wasting of deltoid, biceps and brachioradialis with absent biceps and brachioradialis reflexes on the left. The paraparesis had become markedly worse, especially on the left; bladder function was impaired and there was a sensory level at D10 with proprioceptive loss in the left foot and loss of pinprick and temperature sense in the right leg.

Questions

2. These statements concerning the patient *now* may be true or false:

   (a) Tendon reflexes may be diminished in patients with multiple sclerosis.
   (b) The pattern of weakness and sensory loss suggests an intrinsic spinal cord lesion.
   (c) The findings are still compatible with multiple sclerosis.
   (d) Myelography is now indicated.

Answers

2. (a) **True**
   (b) **True**
   (c) **False**
   (d) **True**

The patient's symptoms and signs have now clearly evolved and suggest a cervical radiculomyelopathy. Although there is a small group of patients with multiple sclerosis in whom tendon stretch reflexes are diminished when the plaque lies in the dorsal root entry zone, they are rare. The pattern of signs in the legs suggests a partial Brown-Séquard (hemicord) syndrome, which occurs more commonly with an intrinsic spinal cord lesion. Only 5% of patients with multiple sclerosis have CSF protein >1 g/l. Myelography is now required to exclude spinal cord compression.

Question

What does this myelogram show (*Figure 1a*)?

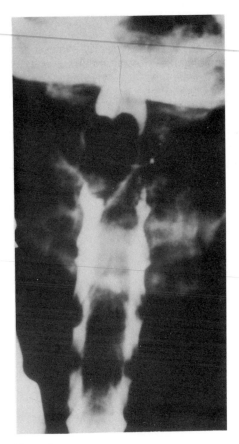

Figure 1a

8

Comment

Myelography showed an extramedullary intradural lesion at C4 on the left. At operation a neurofibroma was removed and postoperatively the patient showed considerable improvement.

Further reading

VICTOR, M. and ADAMS, R. D., 'Disorders of the spinal cord', *Principles of Neurology* (1986), McGraw-Hill, New York, Chapter 27

Case 1.3 Sudden blindness with headache

A 64-year-old miner presented as an emergency to the Ophthalmology Department, having woken blind in his right eye. Three months previously he had become aware of aching and stiffness in the shoulders due, he was told, to arthritis. His symptoms improved after treatment with a non-steroidal anti-inflammatory agent, although he was still aware of some stiffness, both after exercise and on rising in the mornings. As time went by the muscles in his legs began to ache in a similar way and he had difficulty in dressing and in climbing stairs. Headaches developed 4 weeks before admission and, although initially they were mild and localized to the temple, later they increased in severity, being worse when the scalp was touched.

Examination revealed a healthy male. There was no perception of light in the right eye and the pupil was dilated and had no direct light reflex, but the consensual response to light shown in the left eye was normal. Fundoscopy showed generalized pallor of the retina, swelling of the optic nerve head and revealed multiple small haemorrhages in the region of the optic disc. Muscles were tender but there were no other musculoskeletal signs. Palpation over the temples caused pain.

Questions

1. What does the history of aching muscles suggest?
2. What is the probable cause of headaches?
3. Why has this man suddenly gone blind?
4. What investigations are indicated?
5. What treatment should be instituted?
6. What is the prognosis for vision?

Answers

1. Stiffness and muscle pain is due to polymyalgia rheumatica.
2. Cranial arteritis often accompanies (1), causing headache.
3. Occlusion of the ophthalmic artery and infarction of the optic nerve head and retina results from local arteritis.
4. Patients over 55 years with either sudden visual loss or headache should have their ESR estimated.
5. Treatment with corticosteroids resolves symptoms within a very short period of time, usually less than 24 h.
6. Once vision has been lost, prognosis for recovery is poor. Steroids, however, may protect against visual loss in the other eye.

Comment

The patient had cranial (temporal) arteritis presenting with polymyalgia, headache and visual loss. The ESR was elevated at 95 mm/h and symptoms other than the visual loss responded rapidly to treatment with 60 mg prednisone daily. He remained blind in the right eye and within 6 weeks had developed optic atrophy.

Further reading

MEADOWS, S. P., 'Temporal or giant cell arteritis', *Proceedings of the Royal Society of Medicine* (1966), **59**, 329

Case 1.4 Multiple seizures

A 23-year-old woman was admitted to hospital as an emergency after four seizures. She was born normally after an uneventful pregnancy and had an Apgar score of 8/10 at birth. She had a febrile illness treated with antibiotics at the age of 18 months. Intellectual development had occurred normally until this time, but was subsequently delayed and she was educated at a special school. Seizures began at the age of 5 years and were initially generalized; they were poorly controlled on a mixture of primidone and phenytoin. Between the ages of 10 and 18 years her seizure control was relatively good. At the age of 17 years she started to use an oestrogen-containing contraceptive agent and subsequently seizure control deteriorated. Two weeks before admission she had influenza. She lived in a bedsitter with her unemployed boyfriend. There was no history of drug abuse, but she lived in an area where glue sniffing was common.

On examination in the emergency room she was unconscious. Her temperature was 38°C. Her pulse was 120/min and blood pressure 130/90 mmHg. There was no eye opening or speech to pain and she extended all four limbs. Her pupils were dilated and she had normal brain-stem reflexes. She then had two more generalized seizures.

Questions

1. Which of the following should be included in the initial management:

   (a) Measurement of plasma glucose?
   (b) Insertion of an intravenous line?
   (c) Insertion of an airway?
   (d) Administration of intravenous diazepam?
   (e) Administration of intramuscular phenytoin?
   (f) Measurement of serum anticonvulsant levels?
   (g) Administration of oral pyridoxine?

Answers

1. (a) **True**
   (b) **True**
   (c) **True**
   (d) **True**
   (e) **False**
   (f) **True**
   (g) **False**

Two priorities exist in management: firstly, control of the airway and secondly, seizure control. An airway and intravenous access line should be inserted and blood drawn for glucose and anticonvulsant levels (the latter for information about compliance). Seizure control should be attempted initially with one or two intravenous doses of a benzodiazepine, and phenytoin (15 mg/kg) should be given either orally, via a nasogastric tube, or intravenously by slow infusion. Intramuscular phenytoin should not be used because it is not absorbed. Alternatively carbamazepine (400 mg) may be given via nasogastric tube. If bolus benzodiazepines do not control the seizures, then the patient should be admitted to an intensive care unit and a benzodiazepine infusion or intravenous heminevrin or barbiturates may be given. Oral pyridoxine is not needed as pyridoxine-responsive seizures are seen only in neonates.

Anticonvulsants were not detected in her admission blood sample and it was assumed that compliance had become poor following influenza. She had not been investigated previously and needed educating about her epilepsy.

She was treated with a single bolus of intravenous diazepam and carbamazepine via nasogastric tube. Her seizures stopped and she became conscious within 24 h.

Questions

2. Should later management routinely include:

    (a) Skull radiography?
    (b) Cranial computerized tomography?
    (c) Electroencephalography?
    (d) Glucose tolerance test?
    (e) Serial monitoring of serum anticonvulsant levels?

Answers

2. (a) **True**
   (b) **True**
   (c) **True**
   (d) **False**
   (e) **False**

Skull radiographs may show calcification, vault or pituitary fossa abnormalities indicating longstanding pathology. Cranial CT is indicated in patients with focal signs, a focal abnormality on the EEG and those in whom seizures continue despite adequate levels of anticonvulsant. Although the EEG is normal in up to 70% of patients with epilepsy, it may show changes of primary generalized epilepsy (generalized slow wave and spike) or epilepsy of cortical origin (focal sharp waves). Information may also be gained about rarer types of epilepsy including generalized absence epilepsy (3 Hz spike and wave) or focal slow-wave activity suggesting underlying focal pathology. The patient does not have diabetes and a GTT is not indicated. Whereas it is possible to measure the serum levels of most anticonvulsants, a therapeutic range has been satisfactorily established only for phenytoin. In most patients, anticonvulsant level determination is necessary only if they are thought to be intoxicated by the drug, or as a check on compliance.

Comment

Skull radiographs were normal. The EEG showed slow-wave activity associated with some sharp wave transients over the right hemisphere. Cranial CT was normal and it was thought that the patient's seizures were cortical in origin, secondary to childhood encephalitis. She was treated with carbamazepine 400 mg t.d.s. and advised not to drive.

Further reading

MARSDEN, C. D. and REYNOLDS, E. H., 'Neurology' (eds. Laidlaw, J. and Richens, A.) *Textbook of Epilepsy* (1982). Churchill Livingstone, Edinburgh, Section 4

Case 1.5 A forgetful man

A 59-year-old accountant went to see his general practitioner because of deteriorating handwriting. He attended alone and was bemused during the interview, appearing not to grasp what he had been told. There were no focal neurological signs. He was thought to be depressed and was given antidepressants. When these were finished he returned with his wife, who said that he was no longer able to manage his job because of mistakes in simple arithmetic. Once, at home, he had left the gas unlit and twice during the night had been incontinent of urine. There were no other symptoms. He had a moderate concussional head injury 3 years previously (15 min loss of consciousness, 15 h PTA). There was no family history of any similar illness.

On examination blood pressure was 140/95. There were bilateral carotid bruits. He was orientated in time, place and person, but performed series 7s slowly. His forward digit span was four and reverse was three numbers, suggesting that attention and concentration were impaired. He was unable to interpret a proverb in an abstract form. Five min recall and long-term memory were retained. He could perform basic arithmetic quickly and accurately but failed more complex tasks. He was apraxic for imitative movements. Speech and cortical sensation were normal. Sense of smell was normal. Visual acuity was J2 in both eyes and both optic discs were normal. Visual fields were full to confrontation. Upward conjugate gaze was restricted to 25% of normal. There was cogwheel rigidity in the limbs. Tendon stretch reflexes were normal and plantar reflexes flexor. Gait was normal. The jaw jerk was brisk; there were bilateral grasp and palmomental reflexes and a pout reflex.

Questions

1. These statements concerning the physical signs may be true or false:
   (a) Short-term memory is always impaired in global dementia.
   (b) The signs suggested Parkinson's disease.
   (c) Progressive supranuclear palsy may cause this eye movement abnormality.
   (d) The signs may be due to a subdural haematoma.
   (e) Normal gait excludes the diagnosis of normal pressure hydrocephalus.

Answers

1. (a) **True**
   (b) **False**
   (c) **False**
   (d) **True**
   (e) **False**

The clinical problem is to distinguish between an organic dementia and a pseudodementia secondary to depression. In an organic dementia there is always impairment of short-term memory although simple 'bedside' psychometry may not show this in patients of higher intelligence. It is important, therefore, to undertake formal psychometry to demonstrate a discrepancy between verbal and performance IQ and to compare this with pre-morbid intelligence. This patient has a number of more diffuse signs. Cogwheel rigidity is a feature of Parkinson's disease but is also seen in patients who have been given tricyclic drugs. Patients with progressive supranuclear palsy have impairment of both vertical and horizontal conjugate gaze; loss of upward gaze in this patient is probably attributable to normal biological ageing. Dementia is a rare presenting sign of a subdural haematoma and should be excluded in all those with a presenile dementia. Improvement in cognition does not always occur after evacuation of the haematoma. The triad of gait apraxia, urinary incontinence and dementia is not always present in patients with normal pressure hydrocephalus, and a normal gait does not exclude this diagnosis.

Questions

2. What would be the significance of the following abnormalities on investigation:

   (a) Generalized slowing of the electroencephalogram?
   (b) What abnormality is shown on this cranial CT (*Figure 1b*)?

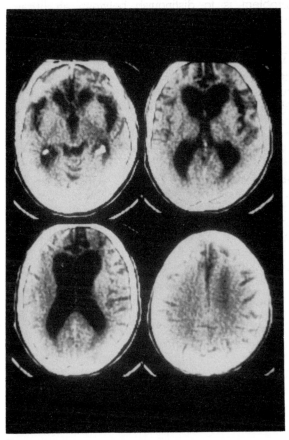

Figure 1b

   (c) A pleocytosis in the cerebrospinal fluid?

Answers

2. (a) In most patients with a presenile dementia the EEG is normal. A focal lesion, e.g. a meningioma or subdural haematoma, may cause lateralized slow (3–5 Hz) waves. Patients with hydrocephalus or a chronic metabolic encephalopathy may have a generalized slow-wave abnormality. Periodic slow-wave complexes sometimes, although not invariably, coincide with myoclonus in patients with Creutzfeld–Jakob disease.

   (b) The principal role of cranial CT in patients with dementia is to exclude a structural lesion or hydrocephalus. Subdural haematoma may be isodense with brain tissue and not visible other than by causing shift of the midline structures. Apart from loss of the cerebral sulci, bilateral isodense subdural collections may not be seen. Patients with Alzheimer's disease may show both ventricular dilatation and prominent cortical sulci – the appearance of cerebral atrophy shown in *Figure 1b*.

   (c) A CSF pleocytosis is rare in demented patients but may occur in those with neurosarcoid, neurosyphilis or other intracranial inflammatory disorders. CSF pressure monitoring may help to detect patients with normal pressure hydrocephalus.

Comment

Psychometric testing revealed a significant difference between verbal and performance IQ and confirmed that the patient was demented, not merely depressed. The EEG was normal and cranial CT showed cerebral atrophy. The extrapyramidal signs were ascribed to tricyclic antidepressants. It was concluded that he had Alzheimer's disease.

Further reading

WALSH, K. W., *Neuropsychology* (1978), Churchill Livingstone, Edinburgh

Case 1.6 An infected tooth

A 20-year-old woman developed left-sided toothache for which she took aspirin and codeine. Ten days later she became febrile and pain spread to the front of the face and the left jaw. The following day she developed a sore throat. Within 48 h pain involved the whole of the left side of the face and she was tender over the maxillary and frontal sinuses. Three days later she became photophobic and was admitted to hospital. Her temperature was 38°C and pulse 120/minute. There was tenderness over the sinuses on the left and the left eye appeared swollen and red. Neurological examination was unremarkable and there was no neck stiffness.

Questions

1. Which of the following should be undertaken:

   (a) Cerebrospinal fluid examination?
   (b) Removal of the infected tooth?
   (c) Drainage of the sinuses?
   (d) Treatment with oral penicillin?
   (e) Treatment with parenteral metronidazole?

Spinal fluid was normal and she was treated with flucloxacillin and ampicillin. Twenty-four hours later she became dysphasic and developed a right hemiparesis. Her conscious level then progressively deteriorated and she was found to have a stiff neck.

2. Which of the following diagnoses should now be considered:

   (a) Hydrocephalus with medullary coning?
   (b) Meningitis with cortical venous infarction?
   (c) Left frontal lobe abscess?
   (d) Herpes simplex encephalitis?

Answers

1. (a) **True**
   (b) **True**
   (c) **True**
   (d) **False**
   (e) **True**

The patient had a dental root abscess which progressed to pansinusitis and orbital cellulitis. Photophobia and blepharospasm can occur as a result of local infection, but as early meningeal spread would also be a possibility, CSF examination would be important. This should have been followed by vigorous treatment of the infection, including removal of the infected tooth and drainage of the sinuses, and the administration of parenteral, not oral, antibiotics including metronidazole to cover anaerobic organisms.

2. (a) **True**
   (b) **True**
   (c) **True**
   (d) **False**

Neurological deterioration occurred rapidly and despite CSF, which initially was normal, it must be presumed that infection has now spread into the cranial cavity. Hydrocephalus may occur when normal CSF drainage pathways are blocked by pus, but this would be unlikely to cause focal signs. Cortical venous thrombosis secondary to infection in the subarachnoid space, cerebral abscess and subdural empyema can all present with seizures, focal signs and a deterioration in the level of consciousness. Herpes simplex encephalitis occurring in this context would be coincidental.

Questions

3. Which of the following investigations is now indicated:

    (a) Repeat CSF examination?
    (b) Cranial CT?
    (c) Electroencephalography?
    (d) Sinus radiography?

Answers

3. (a) **False**
   (b) **True**
   (c) **False**
   (d) **False**

The signs suggest a mass lesion in the left frontal lobe and this should be excluded by cranial CT *before* the CSF is examined. EEG is not the investigation of choice but may show an abnormality over the site of the lesion. Sinus X-rays should already have been done and are no longer indicated as they will add nothing to the management of the patient.

Cranial CT was normal. Slow waves were present on the EEG over the left frontal region; CSF opening pressure was 200 mm, protein 1.2 g/l, glucose 1.8 mmol/l (plasma glucose 4.7 mmol/l) and there were 30 000 polymorph leucocytes/µl. Parenteral penicillin, chloramphenicol and metronidazole were given. The tooth was removed and sinuses drained but despite these measures she died two days later. At autopsy she was found to have pansinusitis and extensive basal meningitis with infarction due to a thrombosed left internal carotid artery.

Comment

Dental and sinus infection is a not uncommon source for intracranial infection. Both the source and the resulting infection should be identified and vigorously treated.

Further reading

WALTON, J. N., 'Diseases of the meninges', *Brain's Diseases of the Nervous System*, 9th edition (1986), OUP, Oxford, 237

Exercise 2

Case 2.1 Dizzy spells

A 38-year-old woman presented with attacks of dizziness. She had always enjoyed good health and while reading Fine Arts at University had taken part in several sports, including badminton and squash. She started running at the age of 28 years. After initially undertaking fairly short distances, she eventually completed a half marathon in 1 h 50 min. While out training she experienced her first episode of dizziness and light-headedness, which was associated with a non-radiating cramp-like pain in the chest. The episode lasted only 3–4 s and she thought no more about it. On a further training run she was again troubled by dizziness and on this occasion lost consciousness for 3–4 s but was then able to continue running and complete her training schedule. She had a further episode while out shopping and was observed to fall to the ground. An eyewitness said that at no time did she convulse and there was no incontinence or change in complexion. Another occurred while she was standing at the bar of a crowded pub, when she was seen to have a generalized convulsion after turning pale and feeling faint. There were no other symptoms and no family history of any similar disorder except that her father died of a myocardial infarction at the age of 48 years. She had three children, all of whom were alive and well.

On examination she had a resting pulse of 45/min; blood pressure was 100/60. There were no abnormal signs on cardiovascular or neurological examination.

Questions

1. What are the possible mechanisms of her collapse?
2. What investigations should be undertaken?
3. What treatment should be given?

Answers

1. Two possible mechanisms exist for these blackouts: either a primary cerebral dysrhythmia, or a cardiac arrythmia with secondary cerebral dysrhythmia.
2. She requires an EEG and a resting and 24 h ECG.
3. Seizures require treatment with an anticonvulsant, e.g. sodium valproate or phenytoin sodium, and advice about driving. Current UK regulations require that she should stop driving for 2 years after the most recent seizure. Any cardiac arrhythmia would also require treatment, e.g. with and/or cardiac pacing.

Comment

Investigations included a normal EEG and resting ECG, but prolonged recording showed bradycardia with episodes of ventricular tachycardia. These resulted in periods of cerebral anoxia with associated seizure activity.

Further reading

ADAMS, R. D. and VICTOR, M., 'Faintness and syncope', *Principles of Neurology* (1985), McGraw-Hill, New York, Chapter 15

Case 2.2 Unexplained coma

A 46-year-old unmarried man who lived alone was found unconscious in bed by his neighbours, who broke into his house when he did not answer the door. At the time of his admission to the Accident and Emergency Department he was drowsy but, to an intensely painful stimulus, he would open his eyes, groan but utter no recognizable words and vigorously flex all four limbs. There was a symmetrical grimace in response to supraorbital pressure. Tone and the motor responses in the four limbs were symmetrical and the plantar responses were flexor. Pupils were equal and reacted briskly to light. Fundi were normal. Eyes were divergent and did not move spontaneously or in response to a doll's head manoeuvre or on cold caloric stimulation.

Questions

1. What is the probable cause of the coma?
2. What investigations are indicated?
3. What other information should be obtained?

Answers

1. The most striking clinical feature about this case is the discrepancy between the level of alertness, as shown by symmetrical flexion of the limbs, eye opening and a groan in response to pain, and the selective depression of the brain-stem function, i.e. loss of eye movement, with preservation of the pupillary reflexes; this combination of signs is characteristic of drug-induced coma. Most drugs causing coma selectively depress the vestibulo-ocular reflexes, resulting in absent oculocephalic (doll's head) and oculovestibular (cold caloric) reflexes, leaving preserved the pupillary reflexes.
2. Blood glucose estimation and a drug screen should be undertaken and the patient observed, to monitor level of consciousness and respiratory function.
3. Friends should be questioned and a careful search made of clothing and house for drugs.

Comment

In this instance, a hospital attendance card was found in his jacket stating that he was attending a psychiatric clinic for treatment of depression. Subsequently, police discovered a number of half-empty tablet boxes in his bedroom, including some containing a tricyclic antidepressant. When the patient regained consciousness he admitted to a suicide attempt by drug overdose.

Further reading

PLUM, F. and POSNER, J. B., 'Exogenous poisons', *The Diagnosis of Stupor and Coma* (1980), F. A. Davies Co., Philadelphia, 241

Case 2.3 A painful arm

A 28-year-old garage mechanic and a workmate were attempting to lift the engine from a car. The mechanic developed severe pain in the neck, radiating to the right side of the face, the right shoulder, arm and chest and followed by a sensation of burning and numbness. He felt unsteady and was aware that objects in his vision were jumping. One year previously he had a similar visual disturbance and since then he had been prone to episodes of vertigo during upper respiratory tract infections. In a coughing bout during the last of these he developed tingling down the inner aspect of the right arm, lasting a few minutes. There was no relevant past medical or family history and he was receiving no treatment.

Examination revealed a fit man who was clearly in pain. The right hand was not sweating. Visual fields were full and fundal examination normal. External ocular movements were full, with downbeat nystagmus in the primary position which became more prominent on looking down. The right pupil was smaller than the left. There was partial right ptosis. The right corneal reflex was depressed and there was loss of pinprick sensation over the right side of the face, neck and arm as far as D4. Speech was normal, but the soft palate elevated towards the right and the tongue was wasted on the left. Tone and power in the limbs were normal. The upper limbs were areflexic; in the lower limbs, tendon stretch reflexes were brisk. Plantar reflexes were flexor and abdominal reflexes absent. Sensation on the left was normal and the patient was able to appreciate light touch, vibration sense and proprioception in the fingers of the right hand. Gait was ataxic. He had a slightly stiff neck and his hairline was low.

Questions

1. These statements concerning the patient may be true or false:

   (a) The signs suggest a lesion involving the cervical roots.
   (b) A low hairline is not likely to be significant.
   (c) A history of an operation for spina bifida would be relevant.
   (d) Symptoms suggest infarction of the medulla.

Answers

1. (a) **False**
   (b) **False**
   (c) **True**
   (d) **False**

The presence of a low hairline and downbeat nystagmus suggests a longstanding developmental lesion at the craniovertebral junction: such lesions are sometimes associated with other aspects of spinal dysraphism, including spina bifida and meningocele which may have been closed at an early age. In addition, the partial XIIth nerve palsy and asymptomatic partial Vth and Xth nerve palsies suggest an intrinsic brain-stem lesion which, during a Valsalva manoeuvre (lifting the car engine) in which intracranial pressure was raised, extended into the upper cervical spinal cord, leading to a dissociated hemicape sensory loss, Horner's syndrome and areflexic upper limbs.

Questions

2. What might these investigations be expected to show:

   (a) Lateral skull radiograph?
   (b) Cranial CT?
   (c) Myelography?

Answers

2. (a) A plain lateral skull radiograph may show basilar impression or a small posterior cranial fossa suggesting a Chiari malformation.
   (b) Cranial CT should be undertaken to exclude associated hydrocephalus.
   (c) Myelography is usually undertaken with prone and supine screening to demonstrate the position of the cerebellar tonsils and distinguish tonsillar descent from other acquired abnormalities such as arachnoiditis or foramen magnum tumours, e.g. a meningioma. Cervical CT myelography may also show contrast within the syrinx giving an indication of its size, provided that it has not collapsed, and also may exclude other lesions such as haematomyelia or an intrinsic cord tumour. Magnetic resonance imaging is the investigation of choice, as it gives most information about the detailed anatomy of the craniovertebral junction.

Comment

Cerebellar tonsillar descent was demonstrated and the patient underwent decompression of the foramen magnum with relief of pain; other symptoms and signs persisted.

Further reading

BARNETT, H. J. M., FOSTER, J. B. and HUDGSON, P., *Syringomyelia*, (1973), W. B. Saunders Co., Philadelphia

Case 2.4 Confusion and focal seizures

A 22-year-old man was admitted to hospital with a short history of headache, confusion and right-sided focal seizures. Three days after treatment with antibiotics for a chest infection associated with fever and rigors, he went back to work. The following day he again felt ill, complained of bifrontal headaches and became confused. His parents thought that he had a recurrence of his chest infection but when his symptoms worsened and he developed twitching of the right arm followed by shaking of the right side of the body he was admitted to hospital. He had bronchiectasis and at the age of 16 years had been considered for a lobectomy. With meticulous care, including postural drainage, physiotherapy and courses of antibiotics, his chest condition had improved and he had been well until the recent infection.

Questions

1. These statements concerning the history may be true or false:

   (a) Focal seizures are unlikely to signify focal pathology.
   (b) The history of bronchiectasis is likely to be relevant.

Examination revealed an ill young man, temperature 39°C. There was finger clubbing. Pulse was 120/min in sinus rhythm. There was a short systolic murmur over the pulmonary area and prolonged rhonchi over the left upper chest. He had bilateral papilloedema with normal visual fields. There was right-sided facial weakness and pyramidal weakness. His neck was stiff, Kernig's sign was absent. The ears and tympanic membranes were normal.

Questions

2. (a) Where do the seizures originate?
   (b) What do the papilloedema and focal signs indicate?
   (c) What is the significance of the stiff neck?
   (d) Would hemianopia be expected with the other focal signs?
   (e) What is the significance of the finger clubbing?

Answers

1. (a) **False**
   (b) **True**

This man has a rapidly progressive neurological disorder and regardless of the presence or absence of focal signs a focal seizure is suggestive of underlying structural pathology. In this instance bronchiectasis might well be relevant since it might act as a source for infected emboli which pass through the heart to cause cerebral abscess.

2. (a) A focal motor seizure is likely to arise from the contralateral frontal region.
   (b) Papilloedema can occur in meningitis or encephalitis due to raised intracranial pressure alone, but the presence of focal neurological signs suggest a space-occupying lesion in the left frontal lobe.
   (c) Neck stiffness without irritation of the lumbar theca suggests a medullary pressure cone due to raised intracranial pressure rather than meningeal irritation.
   (d) A lesion presumed to be in the left frontal lobe would not be expected to produce a hemianopia, as it lies anterior to the optic radiation.
   (e) Clubbing occurs in bronchiectasis and therefore does not necessarily imply an underlying bronchial tumour.

Questions

3. Concerning investigations:

   (a) Is lumbar puncture indicated?
   (b) Would an EEG assist in diagnosis?
   (c) What is shown on cranial CT in *Figure 2a*?

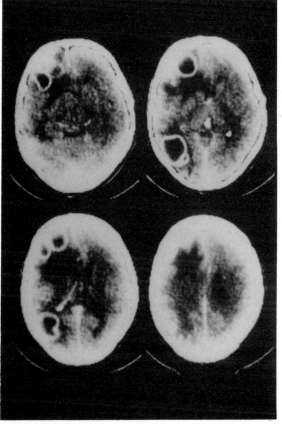

Figure 2a

   (d) Is sputum culture indicated?
   (e) Should examination for fungal material be included?

34

Answers

3. (a) If a space-occupying lesion is suspected, lumbar puncture is contra-indicated as it may cause a pressure cone.
   (b) EEG may show an epileptogenic focus in the left frontal region. A normal EEG would make the diagnosis of herpes simplex encephalitis unlikely (see Case 3.6).
   (c) This cranial CT shows multiple 'ring-enhancing' lesions. Although this appearance can be seen in multiple metastasis or intracranial lymphoma, in this context it is probably attributable to multiple cerebral abscesses.
   (d) This would be appropriate because the same infecting organism may be in both sputum and abscess. Blood cultures should also be obtained.
   (e) Fungal infections including aspergillosis, cryptococcosis and toxoplasmosis may cause an intracranial abscess, especially in patients with diabetes, drug-induced immune deficiency states or those with HIV infection.

He had a leucocytosis of 18 000/µl of which 95% were polymorphs. Changes compatible with bronchiectasis were seen on chest radiography.

Questions

4. These statements concerning the diagnosis may be true or false:

    (a) The presentation is that of herpes simplex encephalitis.
    (b) He has an intracranial abscess which requires surgical drainage.

Answers

4. (a) **True**
   (b) **True**

The differential diagnosis lies between a viral encephalitis and cerebral abscess. Although there is no contra-indication to the use of acyclovir, the clinical picture and cranial CT appearance is that of cerebral abscess and in patients with deteriorating neurological signs or impaired consciousness, or in those in whom the infecting organism is not known, it is customary to drain the abscess surgically. In those who have a stable deficit and in whom the organism is known, it is reasonable to treat with antibiotics and monitor the size of the cavity by serial cranial CT.

Comment

Bronchiectasis is a cause of systemic bacteraemia and septicaemia and therefore a potential cause of cerebral abscess. In this patient the abscess was drained to relieve raised intracranial pressure and yielded a mixed growth of aerobic and anaerobic organisms. He was treated with ampicillin, gentamicin and metronidazole and made a full recovery.

Further reading

STRONG, A. J. and INGHAM, H. R. 'Brain abscess', *British Journal of Hospital Medicine* (1983), **30**, 396–403

Case 2.5 Numb legs on exercise

The managing director of a local engineering firm presented, at the age of 55 years, with a 2-year history of increasing difficulty in walking. Initially, when he walked over half a mile he had pain beginning in his buttocks, spreading, as numbness and tingling, into the posterior aspect of his legs and feet and thence to the anterior thigh and the lower part of the abdomen. There was no significant history of vascular disease. At onset he was thought to have peripheral vascular disease and underwent aortography which showed a normal aorta, internal and external iliac arteries and good peripheral run-off into the legs. Subsequently he was forced to stop walking because of stiffness and aching in his legs, starting after 400 yards. Symptoms were alleviated, within minutes, by rest and partly relieved by bending forwards. On several occasions, after trying to walk off his symptoms, he was incontinent of urine, and it was this that precipitated his referral. There was no past history of disc prolapse or meningitis and there was no significant family history.

Examination at rest was normal. On exercise, when symptomatic, there was weakness in plantiflexion and neither ankle reflex could be elicited. The patient underwent myelography (*Figure 2b*).

Question

1. What is the most probable diagnosis?

Answers

1. The patient gives a history of claudication of the cauda equina which results from an inadequate blood supply to the lumbar roots. This is associated with congenital lumbar canal stenosis or, more rarely, Paget's disease or arachnoiditis following meningitis or myodil myelography. Atherosclerotic occlusive disease of the spinal arteries can also cause similar symptoms, although patients usually have more widespread evidence of vascular disease. An intraspinal structural lesion is unlikely after focal signs have been absent for so long. In lumbar disc prolapse, symptoms are made worse by flexing the spine and the sphincter disturbance is unrelated to exercise. Distal atherosclerotic occlusive vascular disease does not produce proximal symptoms.

Questions

2. What does the myelogram (*Figure 2b*) show?
3. What is the treatment of choice?

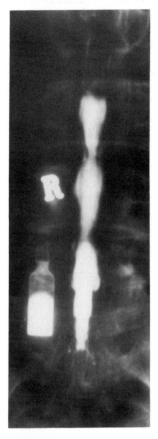

Figure 2b

40

Answers

2. The AP cervical spine diameter at C5 is a measure of spinal canal size (normal range 13–21 mm). Canal diameter in this patient was 11 mm and in the lumbar region the pedicles were close together. Ultrasound examination showed a reduction in the dimensions of the lumbar canal. A myelogram (*Figure 2b*) was technically difficult and showed the wasted appearance of congenital lumbar canal stenosis.
3. There is no medical treatment for this condition. A wide laminectomy to relieve pressure on the cauda equina may help relieve symptoms.

Comment

Lumbar canal stenosis was demonstrated and laminectomy between L2 and L5 relieved the symptoms.

Further reading

WALTON, J. N., 'Lumbar disc lesions and sciatica', *Brain's Diseases of the Nervous System*, 9th edition (1986), OUP, Oxford, 927

Case 2.6 A complicated head injury

A previously fit 60-year-old man went to work in good health. At 10.00 a.m., for no apparent reason, he fell into a pit 12 feet deep. Initially he was rendered unconscious, but on arrival at hospital 40 min later he was conscious but confused. An occipital laceration was sutured and he was given routine antitetanus prophylaxis. No fracture was visible on skull radiography. He was admitted to the observation ward.

On examination he was afebrile with blood pressure 160/90. Distal lower limb pulses were absent. He complained of headache and was confused, disorientated and unable to remember events at home or work that day. His speech contained paraphasic errors and he could not name a simple object. The optic fundi were normal. There was a full range of eye movements. He had a facial and pyramidal weakness with hyper-reflexia and an extensor plantar response on the right. He had a stiff neck and Kernig's sign was present.

Questions

1. The following statements concerning the clinical signs may be true or false:

   (a) The signs suggest that the patient is dysphasic.
   (b) Confusion is due to retrograde amnesia.
   (c) Facial weakness is due to fracture through the petrous temporal bone.
   (d) Neck stiffness and Kernig's sign suggest meningeal irritation due to infection.
   (e) Hemiparesis is due to subdural haematoma.

2. Concerning the head injury the following may be true or false:

   (a) A long period of retrograde amnesia suggests a severe head injury.
   (b) Traumatic subarachnoid haemorrhage may be life threatening.
   (c) Normal skull radiograph excludes a skull fracture.
   (d) There is an increased risk of early epilepsy.

Answers

1. (a) **True**
   (b) **False**
   (c) **False**
   (d) **False**
   (e) **True**

Impaired object naming and fluent paraphasic speech suggest a language disorder. Confused patients often make mistakes in naming but paraphasic speech suggests damage to the superior temporal gyrus – a posterior dysphasia in which comprehension and repetition may also be impaired. Persisting confusion suggests an extending period of post-traumatic amnesia; retrograde amnesia does not cause confusion. Hemiparesis and facial weakness suggest that there is either traumatic damage to the left hemisphere related to cortical contusion or laceration or, less likely, a subdural collection due to tearing of the meningeal vessels. Facial weakness following trauma is discussed in Case 5.5. Meningeal irritation is more probably attributable to a traumatic subarachnoid haemorrhage than to infection.

Clinical evidence suggests a severe closed head injury. Occipital lacerations point to this area as the point of impact, and the period of PTA may extend further.

2. (a) **False**
   (b) **False**
   (c) **False**
   (d) **True**

The length of the period of post-traumatic (antegrade) amnesia is a more reliable indicator of the severity of the head injury than the length of the period of retrograde amnesia. Subarachnoid haemorrhage causing meningism is common after concussional head injury but is not associated with arterial spasm and therefore is not life threatening unless the head injury itself has resulted from the rupture of a berry aneurysm. Conventional radiology does not exclude a fracture through the base of the skull, petrous temporal bone or anterior cranial fossa. Clinical signs including blood behind the ear drum or bruising over the mastoid (Battle's sign), subconjunctival haemorrhages, CSF otorrhoea or rhinorrhoea or an aerocele may suggest a skull fracture. There is also a risk of later epilepsy in those with over 24 h post-traumatic amnesia, early epilepsy, an intracranial haematoma or depressed fracture.

Questions

3. Which of the following is indicated in the early management:
   (a) Serial neurological observation?
   (b) Cranial CT?
   (c) Intracranial pressure monitoring?
   (d) Osmotic diuretics and steroids?
   (e) Anticonvulsants?

Answers

3. (a) Management includes:
   (i) maintenance of the airway and the reversal of life-threatening complications;
   (ii) accurate observation of neurological signs, including level of consciousness using the Glasgow Coma Scale and an assessment of brain-stem reflex activity.
   (b) Cranial CT is generally reserved for those who deteriorate or fail to improve, or who are thought to have hydrocephalus or an intracranial haematoma.
   (c) Management of raised intracranial pressure following head injury is under review. Intracranial pressure monitoring is not widely available and is usually indicated in patients with a haematoma or those who are comatose.
   (d) Intracranial pressure may be reduced briefly with an osmotic diuretic. Steroids have not been shown to be beneficial although widely used.
   (e) Anticonvulsants are indicated after early epilepsy and are often given to those with a cortical contusion or depressed fracture in view of the risk of late epilepsy. The patient should also be advised as regards driving.

Four days after the injury the patient remained confused and dysphasic. Cranial CT showed bifrontal and bitemporal contusions and a small but insignificant subdural haematoma on the left. He remained confused over the next 3 weeks and tended to fall asleep for no apparent reason.

Questions

4. (a) Is he still extending his period of PTA?
   (b) What is the degree of structural damage?
   (c) Is there any reversible pathology?

Answers

4. (a) Patients who remain withdrawn or confused after head
   injury may be extending their period of PTA, or be
   depressed. The EEG would be expected to be abnormal in
   the former, with considerable slow-wave activity, and might
   also show subclinical seizure activity. Depression should be
   treated with drugs rather than ECT which may further
   damage the brain.
   (b) Cranial CT should be used to assess structural damage
   including cerebral atrophy secondary to infarction. Prognosis depends on the degree of infarction.
   (c) Reversible pathology, e.g. hydrocephalus or a subdural
   haematoma, should be excluded.

Comment

He had a severe closed head injury (PTA 3 weeks) with cortical
contusion and traumatic subarachnoid haemorrhage. A subdural
haematoma was shown on cranial CT 3 weeks after the injury.
After evacuation, speech and level of alertness returned to normal.

Further reading

JENNETT, B. and TEASDALE, G., 'Intracranial haematoma', *Management of Head Injuries*
(1981), F. A. Davies Co., Philadelphia, Chapter 7

Exercise 3

Case 3.1 A weak arm after a fight

A man of 21 years, previously in good health, was involved in a brawl with a friend, during which his neck was twisted. Apart from local pain there were no immediate sequelae and there was no sign of external injury. Six weeks later it was noted that his left deltoid was wasted and the patient admitted to sensory loss of 3 weeks' duration over the left shoulder. No action was taken until 2 weeks later when the patient noted weakness at the left elbow and painless sensory loss over the lateral aspect of the forearm and hand. One week later the right hand became weak and he was unable to press on the end of a ballpoint pen with his right thumb. He was a labourer on a hill farm with no relevant past medical or family history.

On examination he was wasted on the left in deltoid, biceps, the wrist and finger flexors, the interossei and abductor digiti minimi. There was a moderate degree of weakness on the left in deltoid, biceps, the long flexors of the medial three fingers, the first dorsal interosseous and abductor digiti minimi. Biceps and finger jerk reflexes were absent. There was sensory loss to a pin over the shoulder and on the lateral aspect of the forearm and medial aspect of the hand. On the right there was an inability to flex the distal joint of the thumb and index finger but no reflex change or sensory loss. The cranial nerves and lower limbs were normal.

Questions

1. Which of the following is likely to account for his symptoms and signs:

   (a) A generalized peripheral neuropathy?
   (b) A mononeuritis multiplex?
   (c) An anterior horn cell disturbance?
   (d) A lesion in the brachial plexus?

2. Which peripheral nerves are involved?

48

Answers

1. (a) **False**
   (b) **True**
   (c) **False**
   (d) **False**

The patchy nature of the deficit, including isolated weakness of the long flexor of the thumb and index finger on the right, suggests a mononeuritis multiplex or, less probably, bilateral brachial plexus disease. In a peripheral neuropathy the weakness is distal and symmetrical. Sensory loss is not found in anterior horn cell disease.

2. The following peripheral nerves are involved:

> left axillary – deltoid, sensation over the shoulder.
> left musculocutaneous – biceps, lateral cutaneous nerve of the forearm.
> left anterior interosseous – wrist and finger flexors lateral three fingers.
> left ulnar – interossei and abductor digiti minimi.
> right anterior interosseous – long flexors thumb and index finger.

Questions

3. Which of the following diseases might account for his symptoms:

    (a) Polyarteritis nodosa?
    (b) Diabetes mellitus?
    (c) Brachial neuritis?
    (d) Lead poisoning?
    (e) Porphyria?

4. The following CSF findings may be true or false:

    (a) Abnormal lymphocytes.
    (b) An elevated total protein.
    (c) A normal opening pressure.
    (d) A normal immunoglobulin content.

Answers

The patient has a progressive painless mononeuritis multiplex which may have a number of different causes:

3. (a) **True**
   (b) **True**
   (c) **False**
   (d) **False**
   (e) **False**

Both polyarteritis nodosa and diabetes mellitus can be associated with a mononeuritis multiplex attributable to nerve infarction. That of polyarteritis is usually painful and associated with eosinophilia and cellular urinary casts. Diabetes should be excluded. Brachial neuritis usually causes plexopathy although it need not be associated with preceding infection or inoculation. Lead poisoning, of which there is no history of exposure, causes an isolated mononeuropathy, often involving the radial nerve. Porphyria normally produces symmetrical polyneuropathy rather than mononeuritis multiplex. Simple partition tests on urine are a relatively reliable screening test for porphyria.

4. (a) **False**
   (b) **False**
   (c) **False**
   (d) **False**

The CSF contents might give some indication of the underlying disease process. An elevated cell count would be unexpected because the disease is thought to lie distally in the peripheral nerves, but abnormal cells might indicate a neoplastic or inflammatory infiltrate. The CSF protein is elevated in patients with a demyelinating neuropathy such as that seen in patients with diabetes or the Guillain–Barré syndrome but would be expected to be normal in patients with an axonal neuropathy or mononeuritis multiplex, as would be the opening pressure and IgG content.

Questions

5. The following findings on neurophysiological study may be true or false:

   (a) Normal conduction velocity.
   (b) Local conduction block in affected nerves.
   (c) Dispersed 'F' waves.
   (d) Abnormal interference pattern on maximal volitional contraction.

Answers

5. (a) **True**
   (b) **True**
   (c) **False**
   (d) **True**

Neurophysiological studies may help to localize the peripheral nerve lesion and show, by electromyography, the extent of denervation and prognosis for recovery. Conduction velocity may be slow in a demyelinating neuropathy but is normal in an axonal, e.g. toxic or paraneoplastic, neuropathy. In severe local lesions a conduction block occurs, but is not a universal finding. 'F' waves represent the discharge of spinal neurones after antidromic activation and are a measure of proximal conduction time. They may be prolonged in those patients with a cervical spondylitic radiculopathy but would not be expected to be prolonged in this patient. A reduced interference pattern on maximal voluntary contraction would be in keeping with a peripheral neurogenic disturbance.

Comment

All haematological and biochemical screening investigations proved unhelpful and neurophysiological studies confirmed the clinical impression of a mononeuritis multiplex. Nerve biopsy was normal. He improved following the administration of steroids and it was thought that his neuropathy was of inflammatory origin.

Further reading

ASBURY, A. K. and GILLIAT, R. W. 'The clinical approach to a neuropathy', (eds. Asbury, A. K. and Gilliat, R. W.) *Peripheral Nerve Disorders* (1984), Butterworths International Medical Reviews, Neurology 4, Chapter 1

Case 3.2 Muscle pain on exercise

A 21-year-old woman gave a 5-year history of pain in the muscles on walking 300–400 yards. She was principally limited by weakness which developed in the muscles of the pelvic girdle. With perseverance she was able to walk the pain off, but after particularly strenuous periods of exercise had noticed that she passed dark-coloured urine. She was well in other respects and there was no relevant family history. On examination there were no abnormal neurological signs.

Questions

1. What type of disorder is this?
2. What are the possible biochemical abnormalities?
3. What investigations are indicated and what might they show?
4. What treatment may assist in reducing symptoms?

54

Answers

1. The history is that of a metabolic myopathy.
2. This may be attributable either to a disorder in the glycolytic pathway or to abnormal mitochondrial function. The first disorder to be described was myophosphorylase deficiency (McArdle's syndrome). This is probably less common than carnitine palmityl transferase deficiency or abnormalities in the cytochrome oxidase system.
3. Electromyography usually shows myopathic changes with low-amplitude polyphasic motor unit potentials. An ischaemic lactate test may fail to show the expected rise in the serum lactate following exercise in patients with McArdle's syndrome. A muscle biopsy with appropriate histochemical stains will identify specific enzyme defects.
4. Glucose loading before exercise may help to prevent pain on exercise.

Comment

The patient had an abnormal ischaemic lactate test with absence of myophosphorylase demonstrated on muscle biopsy. This confirmed the diagnosis of McArdle's syndrome. No biochemical measures alleviated her symptoms.

Further reading

ENGEL, A. 'Metabolic and endocrine myopathies' (ed. Walton, J. N.) *Disorders of Voluntary Muscle* (1981), Churchill Livingstone, Edinburgh, Chapter 18

Case 3.3 A case of involuntary movements

A 75-year-old woman called her general practitioner because of uncontrollable movements of the left arm. She was receiving treatment with haloperidol and benztropine for an agitated depression. Her sister had died 5 years previously from Creutzfeld–Jakob disease and until the time of her death had been cared for by the patient. The patient's involuntary movements began quite suddenly 1 week previously.

On examination she had a smooth goitre. She was in uncontrolled atrial fibrillation, but there were no signs of heart failure. During the examination she had constant fidgeting and posturing movements of the left arm, which were worse on action and which tended to throw her off balance. The tendon stretch reflexes were brisk on the left.

Questions

1. What is the nature of the movement disorder?
2. What anatomical structure is involved?
3. What investigations are indicated?

Answers

1. This is hemiballismus – a continuous 'flinging' movement involving more proximal portions of the limb than does chorea.
2. The subthalamic nucleus of Luys.
3. Electrocardiography to confirm the presence of atrial fibrillation. Cranial CT is usually unhelpful because the infarct is likely to be very small.

Comment

These lesions are usually vascular in origin, presumably in this patient as a result of an embolus as she was in uncontrolled atrial fibrillation. The prognosis for recovery is good and most patients recover within 4 weeks. Tetrabenazine may reduce hemiballismus but can induce parkinsonism.

Further reading

DE BONO, D., 'Do anticoagulants prevent embolism from the heart to the brain?' (eds. Warlow, C. and Garfield, J.) *Dilemmas in the Management of the Neurological Patient* (1984), Churchill Livingstone, Edinburgh, Chapter 4

Case 3.4 Weak legs with incontinence

A 26-year-old man attended the clinic, having become weak in both ankles in the preceding 4 years. He had tripped over kerbs and sprained his right ankle on several occasions. His left side was less severely affected, although ultimately his mobility had been impaired. He had also become increasingly aware of sensory loss beginning in the buttocks and spreading down the back of each leg into the soles of the feet; in the 2 weeks previously the numbness had spread to the dorsum of both feet. He had been impotent for 2 years and, for 8 months, had difficulty emptying his bladder with episodes of incontinence. He was unable to feel the passage of either stool or urine. On questioning he admitted to low back pain from the time of onset of his symptoms. There was no significant family history.

On examination the lumbar spine was normal, there was no pigmentation and no spinal bruits were heard. The muscles of the buttocks and both calves were wasted and there was weakness in dorsi and plantiflexion of the ankle bilaterally. The knee jerks and left hamstring reflex were preserved, the right hamstring and ankle jerk were absent and the plantar reflexes showed no response. There was pinprick sensory loss from the anal margin extending down to the buttocks, down the back of the legs and on to the sole and dorsum of the foot on both sides and to the outer aspect of the shin on the right. The anus was patulous.

Questions

1. The following statements concerning the basis for this disorder may be true or false:

   (a) The findings are those of a bilateral sacral plexus lesion.
   (b) The signs suggest a spastic paraparesis due to a lesion in the dorsal spine.
   (c) The findings suggest a lesion in the conus medullaris.
   (d) The findings are those of a cauda equina lesion.
   (e) A history lasting 4 years suggests a benign disorder and is probably attributable to a central prolapsed intervertebral disc.

Answers

1. (a) **False**
   (b) **False**
   (c) **False**
   (d) **True**
   (e) **False**

The signs suggest that lower motor neurones are involved. Saddle anaesthesia, distal weakness with bladder and bowel involvement is the hallmark of a lesion in the cauda equina. The length of the history suggests a benign lesion such as a lipoma in association with spinal dysraphism, but locally invasive tumours such as an ependymoma can also present with a long history. The lack of acute pain is against a central disc prolapse. Sacral plexus lesions are usually painful and bilateral lesions would have to be very large, or multiple, and are uncommon. Conus medullaris lesions are usually associated with some upper motor neurone signs including an extensor plantar response.

Questions

2. What does this myelogram (*Figure 3a*) show?

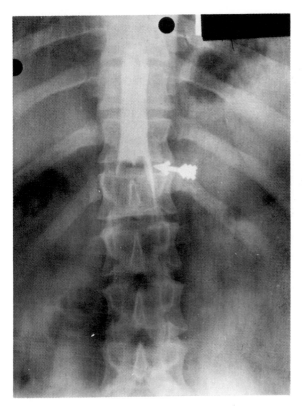

Figure 3a

Answers

2. Lumbar spine radiographs showed widening of the inter-pedicular distance at L4 and L5 with scalloping of the inner aspects of the pedicles at these levels. A myelogram (*Figure 3a*) with introduction of contrast from above showed obstruction to the contrast at the upper border of L1, the appearance being that of an intramedullary conus/cauda equina ependymoma.

Comment

Laminectomy was undertaken to establish both the histology of the lesion and to decompress the lumbar roots. The lesion was found to be an ependymoma and the patient given a course of radiotherapy. The prognosis for this lesion is poor, even with treatment.

Further reading

WALTON, J. N., 'Compression of the spinal cord', *Brain's Diseases of the Nervous System*, 9th edition (1986), OUP, Oxford, 400

Case 3.5 'Febrile' convulsions

A child of 10 years was admitted to hospital after a seizure. She had been born at term and both birth and development were normal. Routine immunizations including whooping cough had been administered and at the age of 5 years she underwent tonsillectomy because of recurrent infections. Two days before the seizure she had felt unwell and gone to bed. The following day she complained of headaches and insisted that the curtains be kept closed. Her mother had not taken her temperature but thought that she had been febrile. On the day of admission she had three episodes of right-sided jerking followed on the last occasion by a generalized convulsion. There was no family history of a seizure disorder.

She looked unwell and was alert but restless. Her temperature was 39.5°C, pulse 140/min and blood pressure 110/75 mmHg. Kernig's sign was present and she had a stiff neck. Optic fundi and horizontal eye movements were normal. Upward eye movements were impaired. She had a mild right hemiparesis with right-sided hyper-reflexia. External auditory meati and the tympanic membranes were normal.

Questions

1. Which of the following diagnoses should be considered:

    (a) Tuberculous meningitis?
    (b) Meningococcal meningitis?
    (c) Herpes simplex encephalitis (HSE)?
    (d) Reye's syndrome?
    (e) A pinealoma?

2. The following statements concerning management may be true or false:

    (a) Intravenous diazepam should be administered.
    (b) Lumbar puncture for CSF examination is required.
    (c) The sinuses should be X-rayed.
    (d) Antibiotics are required.
    (e) Brain biopsy is indicated.

Answers

The history and signs suggest meningeal irritation due to infection and there are focal signs indicating a lesion in the left hemisphere.

1. (a) The history is usually longer in patients with tuberculous meningitis. Seizures and a hemiparesis occur after cortical infarction or rupture of a tuberculoma.
   (b) Meningococcal meningitis may be associated with a rash and often occurs in epidemics in institutions. The diagnosis should be confirmed by bacteriological investigations including cultures from the throat, blood and CSF.
   (c) HSE presents acutely with fever, seizures and focal signs and the diagnosis may be confirmed by finding a rise in serum and CSF viral titres.
   (d) Reye's syndrome (acute toxic encephalopathy with fatty degeneration of the viscera) presents with hypoglycaemia and liver failure following viral infections or ingestion of certain drugs including salicylates and valproic acid. Hypoglycaemia is responsible for focal seizures and signs.
   (e) Although there are focal signs suggesting a lesion in the region of the tectal plate (failure of upward conjugate gaze) which would occur in the presence of a pineal tumour, the other features are those of infection.

2. (a) **False**
   (b) **False**
   (c) **True**
   (d) **False**
   (e) **False**

The signs suggest raised intracranial pressure, and cranial CT should be undertaken before CSF examination. Potential sources for intracranial infection should be examined and these include the sinuses (see Case 1.6). Although brain biopsy can be used to confirm the diagnosis of HSE, diagnosis can be made retrospectively using serum viral titres. Treatment includes that of the seizure disorder and the underlying cause. A single generalized seizure does not require intravenous benzodiazepines, although to prevent further seizures, or further anoxic brain damage, a conventional anticonvulsant, e.g. sodium phenytoin or carbamazepine, should be given. Antibiotics are not required unless pyogenic meningitis can be demonstrated.

The peripheral white cell count was 28 000/μl, and ESR 70 mm/h. Cranial CT was performed.

Questions

3. What does this cranial CT (*Figure 3b*) show?

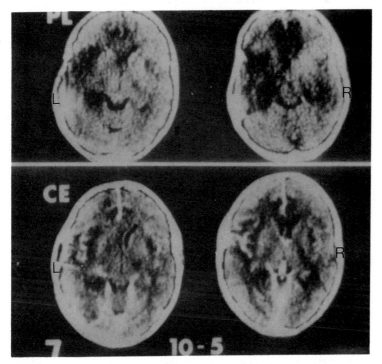

Figure 3b

4. Which of the following measures is now indicated:
   - (a) CSF examination?
   - (b) Carotid angiography?
   - (c) Electroencephalography?
   - (d) Treatment with acyclovir?
   - (e) Administration of antituberculous chemotherapy?

Answers

3. Cranial CT (*Figure 3b*) showed a non-enhancing low-attenuation area in the left temporal lobe with left-to-right shift of the midline structures.

4. (a) This should not be done, because cranial CT showed a mass lesion and there is a risk of transtentorial herniation following lumbar puncture.

   (b) This may give further information about the nature of the space-occupying lesion. In HSE there is a characteristic vascular 'blush' in the infected temporal lobe.

   (c) The EEG in patients with encephalitis may be characteristic (see question 5).

   (d) There is considerable evidence that administration of the antiviral drug acyclovir improves survival of patients with HSE.

   (e) This is not indicated, as there is no evidence of tuberculous meningitis.

Questions

5. What does this EEG (*Figure 3c*) show?

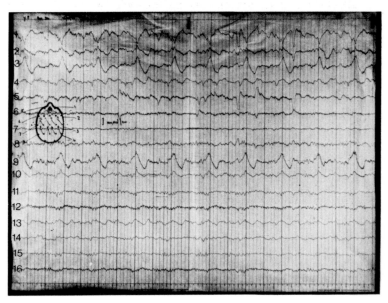

Figure 3c

Answer

5. The EEG (*Figure 3.3*) shows the characteristic lateralized periodic complexes associated with herpes simplex encephalitis.

Comment

Clinically she was thought to have HSE. Lumbar puncture to obtain CSF could not be undertaken because of the intracranial mass effect and she therefore underwent brain biopsy and ventricular CSF was withdrawn at the same time. The CSF contained 10 000 lymphocytes and 500 erythrocytes. The protein was 0.7 g/l and glucose 2.6 mmol/l. No acid-fast bacilli were seen. Immunofluorescent staining of the brain biopsy material was positive for herpes simplex, confirming the diagnosis. She was treated with acyclovir and steroids but continued to deteriorate and died 3 days later.

Further reading

JOHNSON, R. T. *Viral Infections of the Nervous System* (1982), Raven Press, New York.

Case 3.6 Declining abilities in middle age

A 45-year-old housewife was taken to her general practitioner by her husband because of her inability to handle even simple tasks in the home. Three years previously she had become irritable and slightly paranoid; subsequently her memory had started to fail and she had become slovenly in appearance. She could no longer cook or clean the house. Her husband remarked that she appeared to cough in mid-sentence and for 2 years she had been fidgety and was clumsy with her hands. Her past medical history was unremarkable. Little was known about her family history, both parents having died. A maternal aunt was traced and remembered that the patient's father, paternal aunt and grandmother had Parkinson's disease and each had died in a long-stay psychiatric hospital. The patient's only sibling, an elder brother, had emigrated to Australia and was reputed to be well.

General examination was normal. There were no stigmata of chronic liver disease or Kayser–Fleischer rings. There were involuntary movements of the face and limbs at rest, with posturing of the left arm while walking. The patient was demented but language was normal, with no expletives. Speech was punctuated by a series of grunts. The optic fundi and cranial nerves were normal. The only abnormality in the limbs, other than involuntary movements, was the presence of mild cogwheel rigidity. The tendon reflexes were brisk but the plantar reflexes flexor.

Questions

1. The following statements concerning possible diagnoses may be true or false:
   (a) Memory loss occurring in a patient of this age is compatible with the diagnosis of Alzheimer's disease.
   (b) Dementia and fidgeting in this patient suggests the diagnosis of Creutzfeld–Jakob disease.
   (c) Subacute sclerosing panencephalitis (SSPE) may cause this clinical syndrome in middle age.
   (d) This syndrome may be due to Wilson's disease.
   (e) A dominant history of Parkinson's disease suggests that this patient has the parkinsonism–dementia–ALS complex.

2. What is the diagnosis?

Answers

1. (a) **True**
   (b) **False**
   (c) **False**
   (d) **True**
   (e) **False**

The patient has a dominantly inherited progressive dementia associated with involuntary movements. The age of onset, dominant family history and presence of involuntary movements would not be in keeping with the diagnosis of Alzheimer's disease. The length of the history in Creutzfeld–Jakob disease is usually less than 4 years, a family history would be exceptional and myoclonus is the usual movement disorder. SSPE does not develop over the age of 25 years and may be diagnosed on the basis of a high titre of measles antibody in the cerebrospinal fluid. Wilson's disease is one of the few treatable causes of dementia and should be excluded in any patient with dementia and a movement disorder. In Wilson's disease the latter are usually more prominent and the disease tends to present at a much earlier age. Familial Parkinson's disease is uncommon and, in association with dementia and ALS, is usually only seen in Pacific Islands such as Guam.

2. The probable diagnosis is Huntington's chorea.

Questions

3. The following statements concerning this patient's disorder may
   be true or false:

   (a) Grunting during speech is highly characteristic.
   (b) The disorder is of dominant inheritance.
   (c) Cranial CT may show generalized cortical atrophy.
   (d) Senile plaques and neurofibrillary tangles may be seen
       throughout the cerebral hemispheres.
   (e) There is failure of cholinergic neurones originating in the
       nucleus basalis of Meynert.

Answers

3. (a) **True**
   (b) **True**
   (c) **True**
   (d) **False**
   (e) **False**

Chorea affects the muscles of the diaphragm and larynx and causes involuntary grunting during speech. The only true movement disorder other than Huntington's chorea in which grunting occurs is Gilles de la Tourette's syndrome but this is not associated with dementia. Huntington's chorea is dominantly inherited with, usually, complete penetrance. Sporadic cases, i.e. new mutations, do occur. Familial Parkinson's disease is also dominantly inherited, but patients do not show dementia to such a degree. In patients with Huntington's chorea cranial CT may show atrophy of both the caudate head and cortex. Pathological changes are confined mainly to the caudate nucleus in which there is neuronal loss and gliosis; in contrast, in Alzheimer's disease, neurofibrillary tangles and senile plaques occur and there is failure of cholinergic neurones originating in the nucleus basalis of Meynert.

Comment

The notes of other affected members of the family were obtained and it was possible to confirm the family history of Huntington's chorea. Her involuntary movements were partly relieved by tetrabenazine and her children were given genetic counselling.

Further reading

SHOULSON, I., 'Care of patients and families with Huntington's disease' (eds Marsden, C. D. and Fahn, S.), *Movement Disorders* (1982), Butterworths International Medical Reviews, Neurology 2, Chapter 16

Exercise 4

Case 4.1 'Complicated migraine'

A 12-year-old girl had experienced 'migraine' for 3 months. In each attack, lasting up to 12 h, she had headaches and visual hallucinations. A week before admission to hospital her headaches became much worse and she experienced episodes of visual loss on standing suddenly. On examination she had 2 dioptres of papilloedema. The optic nerve was grey and gliotic and there were fresh haemorrhages around the disc. The visual acuity was J2 in both eyes. The blind spot was slightly enlarged. There was a bruit over the left eye. There were no localizing signs and no neck stiffness. She was 65 kg in weight and looked generally alert and well.

Questions

1. What is the probable diagnosis?
2. Name two relevant investigations.
3. What is the prognosis for vision?

Answers

1. The differential diagnosis is that of papilloedema in a girl. Longstanding lesions causing hydrocephalus would be expected to produce an increased head circumference. Posterior fossa tumours including medulloblastoma, pinealoma, pontine glioma, giant cerebellar astrocytoma and ependymoma occur at this age but often cause some restrictions of upward conjugate gaze and a gait disturbance. Benign intracranial hypertension (BIH) is unusual in such a young person, although it can occur in the absence of cortical venous sinus thrombosis or middle ear infection and may present without any other obvious abnormality.
2. CT should be undertaken to exclude a mass lesion; if the ventricles are normal or small in size then it would be appropriate to examine the CSF.
3. The prognosis for recovery of vision, following treatment in patients with raised intracranial pressure, is relatively good, although some patients can lose vision during surgical procedures aimed at reducing intracranial pressure. In BIH, provided that CSF pressure is maintained at physiological levels, the prognosis for visual recovery is good.

Comment

Cranial CT showed small ventricles; CSF opening pressure was >300 mm confirming the diagnosis of BIH. In most patients this goes into remission within 3–6 months and during this time they can be treated either by regular lumbar puncture, or medically with steroids and diuretics. If steroids are contra-indicated or vision deteriorates then thecoperitoneal shunting may be indicated.

Further reading

WALTON, J. N., 'Benign intracranial hypertension', *Brain's Diseases of the Nervous System*, 9th edition, (1986), OUP, Oxford, 140

Case 4.2 Funny turns

A 17-year-old man presented with a 3-year history of 'funny turns'. Attacks had occurred with varying frequency, up to three daily. There were no obvious precipitating factors. Each attack followed the same pattern, beginning with a rising feeling in the stomach. Surroundings appeared unreal and then the patient went into a trance during which he was unaware for about 1 min; subsequently he felt normal. A witness said that during the attack he stopped what he was doing, looked vacant and stared into space making lip-smacking movements. Recovery was rapid and he was able to continue a normal conversation. The patient was otherwise healthy with normal birth and development. At the ages of 1 and 2½ years he had a febrile illness, during each of which he had a convulsion. No abnormality was found on examination.

Questions

1. What is the diagnosis?
2. What is the relationship to the febrile convulsions?
3. What underlying lesion may be found?
4. What management should be recommended?
5. The patient was a delivery boy in a shop, and promotion depended on his holding a driving licence. What action should be taken about this?

Answers

1. Stereotyped trance-like attacks are usually due to seizures. The aura, feeling of unreality and lip smacking suggest partial (temporal lobe) epilepsy.
2. A substantial number of patients with epilepsy have a history of febrile convulsions. Febrile convulsions, of which there may be a family history, are thought to result in anoxic damage, predisposing the patient to further seizures in later life.
3. Mesial temporal lobe sclerosis in Ammon's horn of the hippocampus.
4. It is important to distinguish between primary generalized absence epilepsy and partial epilepsy. An EEG, if abnormal, may show the 3 Hz slow wave and spike pattern of primary generalized absence epilepsy or a focal abnormality in partial epilepsy. Partial seizures may be treated with phenytoin, carbamazepine or sodium valproate. The former has the advantage of being given as a single daily dose. The chance of obtaining complete seizure control in partial epilepsy is about 50%.
5. The patient should be advised as regards the law and epilepsy. The UK Driving Regulations make no distinction between the type of epilepsy or any precipitating factors, and even partial seizures are a bar to holding a driving licence. He is required to advise the DVLC of his medical condition and will not be able to drive until 2 years have elapsed from his most recent daytime (i.e. awake) seizure.

Comment

He was treated with carbamazepine 400 mg b.d. His seizure frequency fell by two-thirds. He was not allowed a driving licence and lost his job.

Further reading

Fitness to Drive (1987), HMSO, London

Case 4.3 Backache and pain in the leg

A 38-year-old bank clerk was well until he attempted to lift a flagstone in his garden. In attempting this his back 'locked': he was bent double and unable to straighten up for 15 min. He remained in pain overnight. When examined the following morning his principal complaint was of back pain radiating into the right buttock and down the back of the leg. Almost any movement made the pain worse; coughing produced an intense shooting pain down the right leg. He had been unable to pass water since the onset of pain although twice he had wished to do so. He had uncomplicated meningitis at the age of 5 years, and was taking ranitidine for postprandial epigastric discomfort attributed to a peptic ulcer. There was no relevant family history.

There was no pyrexia or neck stiffness. There was loss of the lumbar lordosis with left-sided paravertebral spasm. Pain prevented almost all lumbar spine movement, although on attempted forward flexion he developed scoliosis concave to the left. On the right, straight-leg raising was restricted to 20 degrees. The left leg was normal. There was no muscle wasting or weakness. There was loss of pinprick sensation on the sole of the foot. The right ankle jerk was absent. The bladder was initially palpable but he was able to void after adequate analgesia.

Questions

1. The following statements may be true or false:
   (a) There is a lesion in the lumber spine involving the first sacral nerve root.
   (b) The onset of the symptoms suggests a spinal subarachnoid haemorrhage.
   (c) Symptoms are due to a central lumbar disc prolapse.
   (d) Arachnoiditis following meningitis may cause this syndrome.
   (e) Wasting of gastrocnemius and soleus would be expected.

2. The following statements may be true or false:
   (a) Emergency admission to hospital is required.
   (b) Myelography should be undertaken electively.
   (c) The patient should be advised to rest for 10–14 days on a hard bed.

76

Answers

1. (a) **True**
   (b) **False**
   (c) **False**
   (d) **False**
   (e) **False**

The presentation is that of acute sciatica due to irritation of one or more lumbosacral roots, the most common cause of which is a lumbar disc prolapse. Central disc prolapse usually presents with bilateral symptoms, bladder dysfunction, and less pain than a lateral disc prolapse which causes acute sciatica. Spinal subarachnoid haemorrhage may present acutely when straining. Sudden release of blood into the subarachnoid space causes meningeal pain which is usually non-focal and neurological signs are more commonly those of a myelopathy than of a radiculopathy. Because this lesion is acute, wasting in affected segments would not have had time to occur; if wasting were seen in S1, then a more longstanding lesion such as a tumour would have to be considered.

2. (a) **False**
   (b) **False**
   (c) **True**

As only a minority of patients require surgical intervention, the majority of patients can be managed at home with bed rest. If autonomic or motor neurological signs develop, or the pain fails to settle with conservative measures, then myelography should be undertaken with a view to surgery.

Comment

The patient was treated conservatively and the pain settled. He returned to work 1 month later and when examined 2 months later still had an absent right ankle jerk.

Further reading

JENNETT, B. and GALBRAITH, S., 'Prolapsed intervertebral disc', *Introduction to Neurosurgery*, 4th edition, (1983), Heinemann, London

Case 4.4 Positional dizziness

A 36-year-old man presented with a 6-month history of dizziness and unsteadiness. Initially he noticed that any sudden rapid movement of the head was followed by a feeling of rotation. As time went by this became more marked so that bending, turning in bed or standing suddenly would induce the sensation. After 3 months his gait became unsteady and he had increasing difficulty walking in a straight line, tending to bump into objects on the left. For 6 weeks his left hand had been clumsy and he had difficulty in using a fork. In the 3 weeks before admission he had been aware of headaches which were worse early in the morning and he had vomited on two occasions.

Examination revealed bilateral papilloedema and rotatory nystagmus, most marked on leftward gaze. In the limbs, tone, power and the tendon stretch reflexes were normal. He was incoordinate in his left arm and leg and walked with an ataxic gait, tending to veer to the left.

Questions

1. The following concerning his symptoms and signs may be true or false:

   (a) Positionally dependent dizziness is attributable to a peripheral lesion.
   (b) Gait ataxia suggests a brain-stem disorder.
   (c) Incoordination on the left suggests a lesion in the right cerebellar hemisphere.
   (d) Rotatory nystagmus is diagnostic of a cerebellar disorder.

Answers

1. (a) **False**
   (b) **True**
   (c) **False**
   (d) **False**

The symptoms and signs in this patient are diagnostic of a tumour in the posterior fossa causing hydrocephalus. Positional vertigo may occur when either the labyrinth or the central labyrinthine connections are damaged. In peripheral lesions vertigo often develops after a short latency and fatigues, whereas in central disease vertigo is immediate and sustained. Other localizing signs include ipsilateral limb ataxia, and a gait ataxia when the vermis of the cerebellum is involved. Nystagmus itself is non-localizing, merely implying disease of the labyrinth or its connections.

Questions

2. (a) His haemoglobin was 18.5 g/dl; is this significant?
   (b) What does this cranial CT show (*Figure 4a*)?

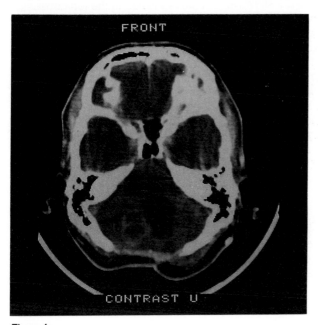

Figure 4a

(c) What associated lesions may be found?

Answers

2. (a) Haemoglobin may be raised in cerebellar haemangioblastoma.
   (b) Cranial CT shows an enhancing lesion in the left cerebellar hemisphere with associated hydrocephalus. The differential diagnosis includes a haemangioblastoma, glioma, secondary deposit and, in younger patients, medulloblastoma, giant cerebellar astrocytoma or ependymoma. In this patient angiography confirmed the presence of a haemangioblastoma which was successfully resected.
   (c) Sometimes these lesions occur as part of the von Hippel–Lindau syndrome. Patients may have retinal haemangiomas, are at risk from subarachnoid haemorrhage from multiple intracranial and spinal angiomas and may also have associated hypernephroma. There is a family history in 20%.

Comment

These patients require extensive screening to find associated abnormalities. Retinal examination of clinically unaffected members may reveal further angiomata.

Further reading

GROSSMAN, M. and MELMAN, K. L., 'Von Hippel–Lindau disease', (eds Vinken, P. J. and Bruyn, G. W.), *Vol 14, Handbook of Clinical Neurology* (1972), North Holland Publishing Co., Amsterdam

Case 4.5 A runny nose

A 55-year-old man was a front-seat passenger in a car travelling at 35 mph when it ran into the back of a stationary vehicle. As a result of not wearing a seat belt he was thrown against the windscreen and sustained a concussional head injury, being unconscious for about 15 min. On admission to hospital he was alert, but confused, and he continued to extend his period of post-traumatic amnesia for a further 4 days.

Two days after admission he was noted to have bilateral subconjunctival bruising. Because of a runny nose he was thought to have developed an upper respiratory tract infection and to avoid infecting other patients he was discharged home. Two days later, when he developed fever and a headache, he was admitted to a neurosurgical unit. Whenever he bent forward he had a profuse nasal discharge. He was fully conscious but had a stiff neck and Kernig's sign was positive. The subconjunctival bruises were resolving.

Questions

1. The following injuries sustained may be true or false:

    (a) A fracture through the petrous temporal bone.
    (b) A fracture through the anterior cranial fossa.
    (c) A traumatic subarachnoid haemorrhage.
    (d) Frontal lobe contusions.
    (e) A subdural haematoma.

2. The following statements concerning the nasal discharge may be true or false:

    (a) It should be tested for glucose content.
    (b) Its presence suggests nasopharyngeal tumour.
    (c) It may safely be ignored.

Answers
1. (a) **False**
   (b) **True**
   (c) **False**
   (d) **True**
   (e) **True**

Fractures through the petrous temporal bone are associated with CSF otorrhoea, bruising behind the ear and blood behind the tympanic membrane; those through the anterior cranial fossa cause CSF rhinorrhoea and subconjunctival bruising. Injury was due to sudden deceleration and probably involved contusions of the frontal and temporal lobes. Tearing of subarachnoid vessels may have occurred but, in the absence of meningism, is unlikely. He is a candidate for a subdural haematoma, although there were no signs to suggest this.

2. (a) **True**
   (b) **False**
   (c) **False**

CSF, unlike nasal secretions, contains glucose. Nasal discharge due to a nasopharyngeal tumour is often blood stained. In this patient CSF rhinorrhoea cannot be ignored and indicates an open head injury. CSF rhinorrhoea often stops spontaneously, but, if persisting beyond 3 weeks, may require surgical closure of the dural defect. During this time patients are at risk from meningitis and air can enter the skull, causing a pneumocele. This may be an asymptomatic radiological finding, but can also cause confusion or a mass lesion which may require drainage. Previously, patients with a compound skull fracture were treated prophylactically with antibiotics, but most units now prefer to adopt an expectant approach.

Comment
The patient sustained a concussional head injury with a fracture through the floor of the anterior cranial fossa resulting in unrecognized CSF rhinorrhoea and meningitis. He was treated with antibiotics and the defect was closed surgically.

Further reading
JENNETT, B. J. and TEASDALE, G., 'Open injuries', *Head Injury* (1982), F. A. Davies Co., Philadelphia, Chapter 8

Case 4.6 Weakness in cold weather

A 43-year-old truck driver was referred for assessment of weakness in both legs which he had noticed while driving during the preceding few months. He had never been a good athlete and had been aware of a slight clumsiness in his hands and a mild degree of unsteadiness in his legs in the previous 2 years. His symptoms were worse in cold weather on winter mornings when he had muscle cramps and he was stiff when trying to get into the cab of his lorry, change a wheel or open the cap of the petrol tank. He had complained of blurred vision for at least 4 years and had passed excessive quantities of urine by day and night for about 6 months. Other than a herniorrhaphy as a child there was no past history. His father had developed cataracts at the age of 45 years and had given up work because of weakness which resulted in his being confined to a wheelchair. A sister had diabetes mellitus and was childless after 23 years of marriage.

Questions

1. Concerning the history the following may be true or false:

    (a) Symptoms may be due to hypothyroidism.
    (b) The difficulties experienced in cold weather suggest polymyalgia.
    (c) The family history suggests a disorder with a sex-linked recessive inheritance.

The patient was thin and had frontal balding. The only abnormality on general examination was the finding of testicular atrophy. On neurological examination he was found to be of normal intelligence. There were bilateral cataracts. Muscles of the face and neck were weak and he had myopathic facies. In the limbs there was gross myotonia on attempted relaxation and percussion myodema was seen. There was a marked proximal weakness and the reflexes were absent.

Answers

1. (a) **True**
   (b) **False**
   (c) **False**

The history is that of myotonia which characteristically is much worse in the cold when patients complain of cramps and muscle stiffness. They are rarely aware of the failure of relaxation which is part of the disorder. Myxoedema can cause similar symptoms (Hoffmann's syndrome) and the TSH level should be measured. In polymyalgia, although stiffness is worst first thing in the mornings, it is not related to the cold. The pattern of inheritance of this disorder is dominant, not sex-linked recessive.

Questions

2. (a) What is the diagnosis?
   (b) What investigations are indicated?
   (c) What treatment is available?

3. The following concerning this disorder may be true or false:

   (a) The myotonia usually causes more disability than weakness.
   (b) There is an association with low intelligence.
   (c) The heart is not involved.
   (d) Bulbar muscles are rarely affected.

Answers

2. (a) Myotonic dystrophy.
   (b) On electromyography the findings are those of denervation associated with high-frequency 'myotonic' discharges. Patients should also be screened for hypothyroidism and diabetes mellitus and examined for cataracts. ECG may show conduction defects.
   (c) There is no cure for this disorder. Phenytoin, procainamide and quinine sulphate may relieve the myotonia. Genetic counselling should be given to affected families.

3. (a) **False**
   (b) **True**
   (c) **False**
   (d) **False**

Clinically, patients with myotonic dystrophy are more disabled by their degree of weakness than by myotonia. This is not the case in patients with congenital myotonia, who tend to stiffen up on exercise but do not become weak. In myotonic dystrophy virtually no proximal muscles are spared and the bulbar muscles are frequently involved. Such a flaccid bulbar palsy may lead to an incompetent larynx and pneumonia. Patients with myotonic dystrophy have a number of associated features including subcapsular cataract, frontal balding, impaired pulmonary ventilation, bone abnormalities and testicular or ovarian failure. In addition there is a recognized association between myotonic dystrophy and low intelligence, and it is the most common neuromuscular disorder to involve the heart, with both conduction defects and a cardiomyopathy leading to heart failure.

Comment

Patients with myotonic dystrophy may not present until their third or fourth decade until weakness has intervened. Unless myotonia is specifically looked for, it may be missed.

Further reading

HARPER, P. S., *Myotonic Dystrophy* (1979), W. B. Saunders, Philadelphia

Exercise 5

Case 5.1 Headache

A 25-year-old woman presented with a 6-month history of repeated attacks of headache. Each was preceded by tingling around the left side of the mouth, which gradually spread over the rest of the side of the face and neck and then, in the next 20 seconds, involved the shoulder, arm and hand. Over the next minute numbness spread like a wave over the trunk. By the time that numbness had spread to the level of the lower thorax the face had recovered; numbness then spread to the left leg and foot and then gradually disappeared. It was associated with a mild degree of clumsiness of the affected part of the body and when the leg was numb the patient was unable to walk. By this time a slight right-sided headache had developed which increased in intensity over a few minutes to become throbbing and severe. The patient would go to bed for about 2 h and on several occasions had vomited. Attacks occurred irregularly but never more than once a week. Between attacks she was well and had no other symptoms. The examination was normal.

Questions

The following statements concerning the disorder may be true or false:

1. A family history of a similar disorder is not relevant.
2. A drug history would be relevant.
3. Cerebral angiography should be performed.
4. Ergotamine-containing compounds are indicated.

Answers

1. **False**
2. **True**
3. **False**
4. **False**

The pattern of these attacks is that of complicated migraine and a family history of migraine is common. Attacks may be precipitated by many different factors including hypertension and pregnancy and the use of drugs such as oestrogens. There is also a slightly increased risk of thrombo-embolic disease in women with complicated migraine who use the contraceptive pill. Further investigation is not usually indicated; very occasionally an arteriovenous malformation may present with complicated migraine but, unless there is a bruit, it is not justifiable to subject the patient to the risks of cerebral angiography. Long-term prophylaxis should be undertaken with drugs such as pizotifen or β-blockers rather than ergotamine in view of the tendency of the latter to cause vasospasm and consequent worsening of the neurological deficit.

Comment

Further enquiry revealed that she had recently started to use the contraceptive pill. Stopping this led to complete cessation of the attacks.

Further reading

BICKERSTAFF, E. R., *Neurological Complications of Oral Contraceptives* (1975), Clarendon Press, Oxford

Case 5.2 A clumsy child

A 3-year-old child was referred because of clumsiness. Six weeks previously his elder brother had chicken pox and 2 weeks later this patient became unwell although no obvious skin lesions were seen. Four days before he was seen he became clumsy and tended to fall when walking or running. His speech was slurred although he remained alert.

On examination he had a trunk and gait ataxia and was mildly dysarthric. Eye movements were full although there was an intermittent and uncontrolled rapid horizontal jerking movement when attempts were made to fixate eccentrically. Limbs were normal apart from an occasional uncontrolled jerk. Tendon reflexes were absent.

Questions

1. What is the diagnosis?
2. What is the eye movement disorder?
3. Name two possible causes of this syndrome.
4. Name two relevant investigations.

Answers

1. This child has infantile polymyoclonia (Kinsbourne's syndrome).
2. Opsoclonus.
3. Following viral infections or in association with a neuroblastoma.
4. Viral antibody titres and urinary vanillylmandelic acid.

Comment

This syndrome usually manifests as a grumpy irritable child who becomes clumsy and falls; other associated features include myoclonus and hyporeflexia. The prognosis for children with the postviral syndrome is excellent and this child made a full recovery in 10 days. In adults the syndrome may occur following a viral infection and as a paraneoplastic syndrome (opsoclonus/myoclonus syndrome) when prognosis for recovery is much worse.

Further reading

DYKEN, P. and KOLAR, O., 'Dancing eyes, dancing feet: infantile polymyoclonia'. Brain (1968), **91**, 305

Case 5.3 Sudden generalized weakness

The day after a 'fun run' a 15-year-old boy was sent to hospital as an emergency because he could not move his legs. He had completed the 13 mile run in 115 minutes by 6 p.m. the day before. At midday he had eaten two chocolate bars and at 7.30 p.m. he had eaten a substantial meal. Because he was tired he went to bed at 9.00 p.m. and slept well but his parents were woken by shouts for help at 7.00 a.m. The patient had woken and was unable to move his legs; he was not short of breath and could speak and drink unaided. While waiting for the family doctor to arrive the patient became unable to lift his hands to his mouth or to sit unaided. On admission to hospital at 9.30 a.m. the patient could only twitch his fingers and toes, although he was breathing normally and could describe the events of the preceding day without difficulty. He had no pain or sensory symptoms.

Questions

1. The following, concerning the differential diagnosis, may be true or false:

   (a) An acute traumatic cervical myelopathy should be excluded.
   (b) CSF examination is required to exclude the Guillain–Barré syndrome.
   (c) He has acute poliomyelitis.
   (d) He has tetanus.
   (e) Myoglobin in the urine would suggest he has a metabolic myopathy.

92

Answers

1. (a) **False**
   (b) **True**
   (c) **True**
   (d) **False**
   (e) **True**

The rapid evolution of weakness following exercise in the absence of sensory loss suggests a metabolic myopathy. The differential diagnosis includes the Guillain–Barré syndrome, and, although excessively rare in the United Kingdom, poliomyelitis. A cervical myelopathy in the absence of trauma and sensory loss would be unlikely and tetanus usually presents with painful muscle spasms related to external stimuli.

There was no significant past medical history. An elder brother and younger sister were well and neither parent had suffered from any neurological illness. The maternal grandfather had been killed at the age of 21 years during the Second World War but the patient's mother was able to recall a story of battle fatigue and weakness before death. A maternal uncle had also suffered from periods of fatigue and weakness throughout school and college life but he had since been well. Another uncle had emigrated to Australia and was said to have episodes of weakness but no further information could be elicited about him.

Examination revealed an alert attentive teenager who gave a full and coherent account of his symptoms. Cranial nerves were normal. He was well muscled. He had a flaccid weakness of all four limbs. Pelvic and shoulder girdle muscles were weaker than more distal muscles. Other than the ankle jerks, tendon stretch reflexes were diminished. There were no sensory abnormalities. Blood pressure was 100/75 mmHg and pulse 40/min.

Questions

2. (a) What is the most likely diagnosis?
   (b) What is the inheritance of this disorder?
   (c) What treatment would be expected to improve his condition?
   (d) What is the prognosis?
   (e) What measures should be recommended to prevent a recurrence?

Answers

2. (a) Hypokalaemia due either to periodic paralysis, drugs or Conn's syndrome is the most likely cause of this acute myopathy. Myasthenia, thyrotoxicosis and porphyria should also be excluded. Thyrotoxic periodic paralysis usually only occurs in Chinese and Malays.
   (b) The history of weakness in the mother's family is likely to be relevant and suggests a familial periodic paralysis; occasionally females do not manifest the disease.
   (c) Hypokalaemia should be treated with 10 g potassium chloride by mouth followed by a further 5 g should recovery be delayed.
   (d) Total paralysis including that of the respiratory muscles is rare: attacks usually resolve completely within 6–24 h. Symptoms often first become manifest during the second decade, worsening throughout the third and then stopping; however, a significant number of patients may go on to develop a myopathy with resulting proximal weakness.
   (e) Prophylaxis includes potassium supplements and a low-carbohydrate low-salt diet. Excessive exercise should be avoided.

Investigations revealed serum potassium 2.0 mmol/l; other electrolytes were normal. ECG showed prominent U waves with flattened T waves and prolongation of the PR interval.

Comment

He came from a family with hypokalaemic periodic paralysis. With oral potassium his weakness recovered and he remained attack-free on the regime described in answer 2(e).

Further reading

ENGEL, A., 'Metabolic and endocrine myopathies', (ed. J. N. Walton), *Disorders of Voluntary Muscle*, 4th edition (1981), Churchill Livingstone, Edinburgh, Chapter 18

Case 5.4 Tingling fingers and toes

A 67-year-old retired labourer had tingling in his fingers and toes. This had become progressively more disabling over the preceding 2 months, during which time his hands had become weak. He was also aware of tight band-like sensations in his legs and feet and complained of difficulty in walking, which he attributed to unsteadiness and a tendency to catch his feet. Exercise made his symptoms worse. He had developed urgency and frequency of micturition during this time and also thought that he had become more constipated than usual. He had been impotent for 2 years. He had been treated with diuretics for mild hypertension for 20 years, and had complained of backache since starting work. This had been treated from time to time with physiotherapy and manipulation.

Blood pressure was 130/90 mmHg. Pulse rate was 72/min, in sinus rhythm. There was loss of the cervical and lumbar lordosis and cervical spine movement was limited by pain. Cranial nerve examination was normal. There was reduced pinprick sensation over both hands and forearms. Biceps and forearm muscles were wasted and he was weak in biceps, brachioradialis, wrist flexors and extensors and the intrinsic muscles of the hands. Tone was increased in both legs and there was weakness in hip and knee flexion and in dorsiflexion. Other muscles were of normal strength. There was sensory loss to a tuning fork below the costal margin and loss of proprioception at the toes and ankles. The jaw jerk was normal. Biceps and brachioradialis reflexes were absent with inversion to the finger jerks. All lower limb tendon stretch reflexes were pathologically brisk with associated ankle and knee clonus. Plantar reflexes were extensor.

Questions

1. The following causes of the symptoms and signs may be true or false:

   (a) A mixed sensorimotor neuropathy.
   (b) Vitamin B_{12} deficiency.
   (c) Cervical cord compression.
   (d) A central cord syndrome

Answers

1. (a) **False**
   (b) **False**
   (c) **True**
   (d) **False**

The signs are those of a cervical radiculomyelopathy. Absent reflexes in the upper limbs suggest focal disease at the C5/6 level rather than a peripheral neuropathy. Vitamin B_{12} deficiency (subacute combined degeneration of the cord) may begin in the upper limbs although usually the signs include absent tendon reflexes with extensor plantar responses. A central cord syndrome would be associated with a dissociated sensory loss in a cape or hemicape distribution.

Questions

2. Concerning investigation, the following may be true or false:

   (a) Nerve conduction studies would indicate the site of the lesion.
   (b) Radiographs of the cervical spine are indicated.
   (c) Lumbar radiculography is the investigation of choice.

3. Concerning treatment, the following may be true or false:

   (a) A cervical collar is sufficient.
   (b) Foraminotomy is the surgical treatment of choice.
   (c) Spasmolytics are indicated.

Answers

2. (a) **True**
   (b) **True**
   (c) **False**

Investigations are indicated to confirm the site of cord compression. These include plain radiographs of the cervical spine to show degenerative disease and to estimate the size of the spinal canal, and a cervical myelogram to show the extent of intraspinal disease. Lumbar radiculography is not indicated. Nerve conduction studies would be expected to show normal conduction velocities in the limbs but delayed 'F' wave latencies (Case 3.1) in the cervical region.

3. (a) **False**
   (b) **False**
   (c) **True**

There is not universal agreement about the place of surgery in patients with a cervical spondylotic radiculomyelopathy. If there is rapid deterioration in lower limb function due to cord compression, then surgery (either by anterior discectomy or posterior laminectomy) may halt the deterioration. Foraminotomy may be effective in reducing root symptoms in the arms. Spasticity should be treated with a spasmolytic such as baclofen or dantrolene sodium. A cervical collar is not generally indicated, except postoperatively.

Comment

Myelography demonstrated a single anterior cervical disc protrusion at C4/5. An anterior discectomy with foraminotomy relieved the spinal cord compression and reduced sensory symptoms in the arms.

Further reading

MONRO, P., 'What has surgery to offer in cervical spondylosis'. (eds Warlow, C. and Garfield, J.), *Dilemmas in the Management of the Neurological Patient* (1984), Churchill Livingstone, Edinburgh, 168

Case 5.5 Dizziness after going to a discothèque

A 19-year-old man left a discothèque at 1.30 a.m. after 3 pints of beer. He slipped on the edge of the pavement and knocked the back of his head on the kerb. He was unconscious for 2–3 minutes but had no significant period of retrograde amnesia. He complained, in the Accident and Emergency Department, of intense dizziness and was noted by the casualty officer to have nystagmus. He was assumed to be drunk and was sent home. Twenty-four hours later he returned because of persisting dizziness, regardless of head position, and deafness. On examination there was a bruise behind the right ear but no visible blood behind the tympanic membrane. He had nystagmus with the fast phase to the left on left lateral gaze. The amplitude of the nystagmus appeared to increase with the eyes closed on palpating the globe. He was deaf on the right. Examination of the remainder of the cranial nerves was normal.

One week later he developed a right-sided facial weakness; tearing and taste were preserved.

Questions

1. Which of the following may account for his vertigo and nystagmus:

   (a) Alcohol?
   (b) Labyrinthine haemorrhage?
   (c) Brain stem haematoma?
   (d) Menière's disease?
   (e) Multiple sclerosis?

2. Which of the following may be the cause of the deafness:

   (a) Traumatic damage to the auditory nerve or cochlea?
   (b) Disruption of the ossicular chain?
   (c) A brain-stem injury?

Answers

1. (a) **False**
   (b) **True**
   (c) **False**
   (d) **False**
   (e) **False**

The description of the nystagmus suggests a peripheral lesion with the fast phase always in the same direction and an amplitude which increases when fixation is abolished. This occurs after trauma when there is a haemorrhage into the labyrinth associated with a fracture through the petrous temporal bone (as evidenced in this case by the presence of Battle's sign). The history is not that of Menière's disease. Nystagmus of central origin, e.g. in alcohol poisoning, brain-stem haematoma or multiple sclerosis, is usually present on lateral gaze to each side with the fast phase in the direction of gaze.

2. (a) **True**
   (b) **True**
   (c) **False**

Unilateral deafness following trauma may be due either to damage to the cochlea or auditory nerve, or may follow disruption of the ossicular chain. Audiometric testing is needed to distinguish the two, and the latter may require surgical repair. Deafness due to brain-stem disease is extraordinarily rare.

Questions

3. The following statements concerning the facial palsy may be true or false:

   (a) Its occurrence is coincidental.
   (b) It is the result of trauma to the facial nerve.
   (c) Lacrimation would be absent with a lesion in the facial canal.
   (d) The site of the lesion is likely to be proximal to the origin of the corda tympani.
   (e) The prognosis for recovery is likely to be good.

Answers

3. (a) **False**
   (b) **True**
   (c) **False**
   (d) **False**
   (e) **True**

Two types of facial nerve injury may occur after trauma to the petrous temporal bone. The VIIth nerve may be subject to immediate neuropraxia, neurotmesis or axonotmesis in the bony canal at the time of injury, or swelling may occur up to 10 days later, causing a delayed facial palsy. The prognosis for recovery in the latter is good. Loss of lacrimation occurs only when the lesion lies in the subarachnoid space, because the petrosal nerve to the lacrimal gland leaves the facial nerve before it enters the facial canal. In this patient, as taste was preserved, the nerve is likely to have been damaged distally within the canal after the origin of the corda tympani.

Comment

This patient sustained a fracture through the petrous temporal bone with haemorrhage into the semicircular canals. The ossicular chain was disrupted and required surgical reconstruction. The facial palsy recovered in 4 weeks.

Further reading

CARTLIDGE, N. E. F. and SHAW, D. A. 'Facial nerve injuries', *Head Injury* (1981), W. B. Saunders, Philadelphia, 68

Case 5.6 False localizing signs?

A 44-year-old woman, previously in good health, had become deaf over a 3-month period. She consulted her general practitioner because of hazy vision and admitted to occasional waking headaches. The following week the left side of her face became numb and she experienced double vision on looking to the right. Twice she had a profuse clear nasal discharge which settled spontaneously. There was no history of head injury. She had had two normal pregnancies and was pre-menopausal.

Higher cerebral function was normal. She was anosmic. Visual acuity was J2 in each eye and there was bilateral haemorrhagic papilloedema with 2 dioptres disc swelling and gliosis around the optic disc. She had an incongruous left homonymous hemianopia with a larger right-sided nasal field defect. Pupillary reflexes were normal. There was bilateral failure of abduction of the eyes with loss of upward vertical conjugate gaze. Pinprick sensation was absent over the left side of the face in all divisions of the trigeminal nerve. There was mild bilateral sensorineural deafness. VIIth, Xth, XIth and XIIth cranial nerves were normal. Tendon stretch reflexes in the limbs were pathologically brisk, there was a pout and left-sided palmomental and grasp reflex. The remainder of the neurological examination was normal.

Questions

1. The following concerning the localizing value of the physical signs may be true or false:

   (a) Anosmia suggests a lesion in the temporal lobe.
   (b) Raised intracranial pressure has been present for a long time.
   (c) The visual field defect suggests a lesion in the optic tract.
   (d) The eye movement disorder suggests a lesion in the tectal plate.
   (e) The eye movement disorder suggests a lesion in the medial longitudinal fasciculus.
   (f) Facial sensory loss and deafness suggests a lesion in the cerebellopontine angle.
   (g) Unilateral grasp and palmomental reflexes suggest diffuse cerebral disease.

Answers

1. (a) **False**
   (b) **True**
   (c) **True**
   (d) **True**
   (e) **False**
   (f) **False**
   (g) **False**

The patient has longstanding raised intracranial pressure as evidenced by gliotic papilloedema and failure of upward vertical conjugate gaze due to pressure on the tectal plate; the question is, which of the other signs is localizing and which false localizing? Generally, in patients such as this, signs of supratentorial origin, e.g. the field defect and lateralized primitive reflexes, are of localizing value and those of infratentorial origin, e.g. facial sensory loss, bilateral VIth and VIIIth nerve palsies, are not. Anosmia may occur when the olfactory nerve is damaged, e.g. due to a subfrontal meningioma or following trauma, or may accompany the common cold or the use of drugs such as penicillamine but is not seen in temporal lobe disease. The latter may cause a paraosmia or olfactory hallucination of a partial seizure.

Questions

2. Which of the following should be included in the differential diagnosis?

   (a) Benign intracranial hypertension?
   (b) Carcinomatous meningitis?
   (c) Acoustic neuroma?
   (d) Intraventricular meningioma?
   (e) Subfrontal meningioma?

Answers

2. (a) **False**
   (b) **True**
   (c) **False**
   (d) **True**
   (e) **True**

The majority of signs are extraparenchymal and, for the reasons given above, suggest a lesion in the supratentorial compartment, e.g. an intraventricular or subfrontal meningioma. Carcinomatous meningitis might cause this number of apparent cranial nerve palsies but would be unlikely to cause such longstanding papilloedema. Patients with benign intracranial hypertension may have one, or occasionally more than one, false localizing sign but rarely as many as in this patient. Acoustic neuroma would not, unless bilateral, usually present with bilateral hearing loss.

Comment

Cranial CT showed a large right-sided intraventricular meningioma which was successfully resected. Two days later the patient's sense of smell and hearing had returned to normal. Facial sensation and the ophthalmoplegia resolved by the time of discharge, suggesting that all of these were false localizing signs.

Further reading

GASSEL, M. M., 'False localising signs (A review of the concept and analysis of the occurrence in 250 cases of intracranial meningioma)', *Archives of Neurology and Psychiatry (Chicago)*, (1961), **4**, 526

Exercise 6

Case 6.1 What am I doing here?

A 64-year-old sheet metal worker was noted to be confused at work. By the time that he arrived in the Accident and Emergency Department he had recovered but had no recollection of preceding events. He left home, as usual, at 8.15 a.m. and arrived at work at 9.05 a.m. He worked on his bench until 11.00 a.m. when, at break, workmates thought his behaviour was normal. At lunch 2 h later friends thought that his behaviour was strange. After lunch he was unable to find his way back to work and kept repeating 'What am I doing here; who are you?' and similar phrases. The works medical officer called to see the patient and thought him to be confused and sent him to the Accident and Emergency Department.

On arrival the patient claimed to be normal, although he was amnestic for events between 11.00 a.m. and 2.30 p.m. Formal testing confirmed normal memory and orientation. Blood pressure was 160/100 mmHg. There were no bruits.

Questions

1. What is the differential diagnosis?
2. What investigations are indicated?
3. Is treatment required?
4. What is the prognosis?

Answers

1. This is most likely to be transient global amnesia (TGA); the differential diagnosis includes hypoglycaemia secondary to insulinoma, a prolonged complex partial seizure or hysterical fugue. Hypoglycaemic attacks are usually relatively short and accompanied by adrenergic symptoms. Hysterical symptoms should not be seriously considered in a male over the age of 50.
2. Screening tests for vascular disease, a 48 h fast and EEG.
3. No specific treatment is required; advice should be given with regard to control of blood pressure and smoking. No strict policy with regard to driving can be outlined although it would seem wise to restrict the patient for a few months,
4. The prognosis is good; most patients rarely have more than one TGA. When multiple attacks occur the diagnosis is usually that of a seizure disorder.

Comment

TGA is a form of transient ischaemic attack occurring in the distribution of the posterior cerebral artery, affecting the medial aspect of the temporal lobes. Attacks are characterized by a period of transient confusion lasting up to a few hours during which time patients appear to be confused and disorientated and fail to make new memory. Patients may continue with complex activities including work and driving but at the end of the attack will be amnestic for events occurring during the period of apparent confusion.

Further reading

HEATHFIELD, K. W. G., CROFT, P. B. and SWASH, M., 'The syndrome of transient global amnesia', *Brain* (1973), **96**, 729

Case 6.2 Repeated attacks of pain in the eye

A 30-year-old man had a history of episodes of pain in and around the left eye. His first attack was at the age of 21 years when he was woken at 2.00 a.m. with a burning pain in the left eye. It increased in severity over a few minutes causing him to get out of bed and walk around the room. After 30 min the pain began to diminish and it disappeared completely after 45 min. A similar pain caused him to wake every night for the next 2 weeks. He then remained pain free for 5 years, when he had similar attacks over a 4-week period. The present series of attacks had begun 1 week previously and were again similar in character although longer in duration. He had up to three attacks each night and during them the eye watered. There was no past medical history. Neurological examination was normal.

Questions

1. What is the diagnosis?
2. What investigations are indicated?
3. What treatment should be offered?

Answers

1. Periodic migrainous neuralgia (cluster headaches).
2. In the absence of physical signs no investigations are needed. Cranial CT and carotid angiography are indicated if there is an associated pupillary or eye movement disorder to exclude a lesion in or around the cavernous sinus.
3. A β-blocker or methysergide given prophylactically will often abort attacks. Long-term treatment with the latter should be avoided because of the risk of retroperitoneal fibrosis. Patients with nocturnal attacks may find ergotamine by suppository beneficial if used before retiring. In resistant cases, or those patients with chronic cluster headaches, lithium carbonate or indomethacin may be of use. Individual attacks are short and self-limiting and do not require treatment unless very severe, when breathing 100% oxygen early in the attack may lessen the severity of the pain.

Comment

Periodic migrainous neuralgia is thought to be a form of migraine. It typically affects young men. Stereotyped attacks of unilateral pain in the eye occur at the same time of day, lasting 1–2 h for up to 4–6 weeks. Pain may be associated with epiphora and nasal congestion.

Further reading

VICTOR, M. and ADAMS, R. D., 'Headache and other craniofacial pains', *Principles of Neurology* (1986), McGraw-Hill, New York, Chapter 7

Case 6.3 A wet bed

A 31-year-old man sought medical advice because of nocturnal incontinence. Four times in the previous year he had woken in the morning in a wet bed, having been incontinent of urine. Each time he had gone to bed feeling well, having taken neither drugs nor an excessive quantity of alcohol. Bladder function during the day was normal. Two years previously he had sustained a mild concussional head injury in a road traffic accident in which he remembered the car skidding and then nothing more until arriving in the hospital X-ray department. Examination was normal.

Questions

1. What is the probable diagnosis?
2. What is the underlying cause?
3. What investigations are indicated?

Answers

1. Nocturnal epilepsy. Incontinence occurs when bladder capacity is exceeded and there is impairment of sphincter control. When incontinence does not rouse the patient from sleep it is likely that there is loss of consciousness or awareness. This, in combination with lack of sphincter disturbance during the day, suggests that the incontinence is due to a seizure disorder.
2. A previous head injury may be relevant; however, the risk of epilepsy following a concussional head injury with PTA less than 24 h when there has been no early epilepsy or focal cortical damage is small (1%). Seizures developing in an adult require investigation, because up to 20% will have focal intracranial disease, e.g. a tumour.
3. Investigations are those for a seizure disorder including skull and chest radiography, EEG and cranial CT.

Comment

EEG showed a right frontal slow-wave focus and cranial CT confirmed the presence of a low-attenuation contrast-enhancing lesion which, on biopsy, was found to be an astrocytoma.

Further reading

LAIDLAW, J. and RICHENS, A., 'Pathology and pathophysiology', *A Text Book of Epilepsy* 2nd edition, (1981), Churchill Livingstone, Edinburgh, Chapter 11

Case 6.4 A painful hand

A 62-year-old right-handed miner presented with a 3-month history of pain of an increasingly severe nature in the left arm. Symptoms had started as an ache in the elbow, followed by painful pins and needles from the elbow extending down the forearm to the tips of the little and ring fingers. There had also been a gradual loss of dexterity with the hand, such that opening doors or turning a tap was impossible. Touching the hand caused exquisite pain and he protected it constantly. Sleep was disturbed by the pain and there was no position which gave him any relief. Two years previously he had a myocardial infarction followed by pain in the left shoulder and a stiff arm lasting 6 months. He smoked 20 cigarettes daily and drank 2–4 pints of beer weekly.

Questions

1. The following sites of origin of the pain may be true or false:

   (a) The ulnar nerve in the olecranon groove.
   (b) The Vth and VIth cervical roots.
   (c) The anterior interosseous nerve in the pronator tunnel.
   (d) The sympathetic outflow at T1.
   (e) The spinal grey matter.

Answers

1. (a) **False**
   (b) **False**
   (c) **False**
   (d) **True**
   (e) **True**

The distribution and character of the pain is suggestive of a lesion in the brachial plexus, lower cervical roots or central grey matter of the spinal cord. A compressive ulnar neuropathy may be painful but rarely is it so severe and usually does not involve the entire forearm. The distribution is not that of the C5 or C6 root and the anterior interosseus nerve has no sensory branches.

On examination he was a thin, emaciated man who looked unwell and was in obvious pain. There was a partial left ptosis with meiosis of the pupil. Sweating was absent over the left side of the face. The left hand was dry, red and shiny with wasting of the interossei, thenar and hypothenar muscles. Both ulnar nerves were palpable but not tender. There was a flexion contracture of the fingers, although the hand was otherwise hypotonic. Gentle stroking of the skin over the ring and little fingers caused severe pain and sensory loss to all modalities was detected over the palmar and dorsal aspects of the hand and the medial side of the forearm below the elbow. The intrinsic muscles and finger extensors on the left were weak. Tendon stretch reflexes other than the left finger flexor reflex were preserved.

Questions

2. The following concerning the physical signs may be true or false:

   (a) The distribution of the sensory loss suggests a lesion in the ulnar nerve.
   (b) Ptosis and pupillary abnormality suggests a lesion at C8.
   (c) Wasting and weakness in the thenar muscles suggests a lesion at T1.
   (d) The appearance of the hand suggests involvement of autonomic fibres.
   (e) An absent finger flexor reflex indicates a lesion at C5.

3. What is the diagnosis?

4. Which of the following would be the investigation of choice:

   (a) Nerve conduction studies?
   (b) Oblique radiographs of the cervical spine?
   (c) Chest radiography?
   (d) CT myelography?

Answers

2. (a) **False**
   (b) **False**
   (c) **True**
   (d) **True**
   (e) **False**

A Horner's syndrome (ptosis, meiosis and loss of sweating on the face) and absence of sweating in the hand suggests a lesion in the sympathetic outflow at T1. The motor signs and sensory loss reflect a lesion in the C8/T1 roots. Sensory loss is greater than would be expected in an ulnar nerve lesion. Finger flexion is a C8 reflex.

3. Pancoast tumour infiltrating cervical roots or brachial plexus.

4. (a) **False**
   (b) **False**
   (c) **True**
   (d) **False**

Diagnosis is confirmed if a chest radiograph shows an apical lesion with erosion of the first rib. Oblique views of the cervical spine may show enlargement of the intervertebral foraminae and bony destruction. CT myelography may demonstrate the extent of the tumour if radical surgical excision was planned. Distal conduction velocities would be expected to be normal; proximal latency ('F' wave latency) might be prolonged, suggesting involvement of the nerve roots. Electromyography would show denervation in affected muscles.

Comment

ESR was 60 mm/h and chest radiography showed a lesion in the apex of the left lung with erosion of the first rib. A Pancoast tumour may invade the lower cervical roots, sympathetic outflow and brachial plexus, causing severe dysaesthetic pain and C8 T1 motor signs. Radiotherapy and carbamazepine may assist with pain relief.

Further reading

KORI, S. H., FOLEY, K. M. and POSNER, J. B., 'Brachial plexus lesions in patients with cancer: 100 cases', *Neurology (NY)* (1981), **31**, 45–50

Case 6.5 Blank spells

A man aged 56 years, a natural Gaelic speaker from the Outer Hebrides, attended with his wife because of frequent episodes of confused behaviour. These consisted of an olfactory hallucination, nausea, a sense of doom and sudden cessation of speech. He had never lost consciousness or had a generalized convulsion. He had suffered from non-specific headaches for many years and in one of these had vomited profusely. He shaved less than previously and had been impotent for 10 years. His weight was stable and there had been no change in body habitus. He had no particular preference for warm or cold weather and there was no dizziness on standing. There was no significant past medical or family history. He smoked a pipe and drank socially. He worked as an accountant and had recently returned from a trip to India.

On examination he was clean shaven and had a dry skin. Blood pressure was 140/90 mmHg. There were bilateral carotid bruits. He had gynaecomastia with galactorrhoea to expression. Genitalia were normal. Neurological examination revealed a small upper left monocular temporal quadrantanopia, a pout reflex, and a right palmomental and grasp reflex.

Questions

1. Which of the following may be responsible for his visual failure:

   (a) Previous retrobulbar neuritis?
   (b) Pituitary tumour?
   (c) Sphenoidal wing meningioma?
   (d) Tobacco amblyopia?
   (e) Central retinal artery occlusion?

118

Answers

1. (a) **False**
   (b) **True**
   (c) **True**
   (d) **False**
   (e) **True**

The presence of a monocular visual field defect suggests a lesion inferiorly and medially to the optic nerve at the level of the optic chiasm, which may be either a pituitary tumour or, less probably, a sphenoidal wing meningioma. Retrobulbar neuritis or tobacco amblyopia would produce optic atrophy with a central scotoma; although a central retinal artery occlusion may produce a similar field defect, it is usually associated with local changes which are visible on fundoscopy.

Questions

2. What is the significance of the following symptoms and signs:

   (a) Speech arrest, nausea and a sense of doom?
   (b) The need to shave less frequently?
   (c) Impotence?
   (d) Galactorrhoea to expression?
   (e) Unilateral palmomental reflex?

3. Which of the following investigations is indicated:

   (a) Serum 11-hydroxycorticosteroid estimation?
   (b) Serum prolactin estimation?
   (c) Lateral skull radiograph?
   (d) Carotid angiogram?
   (e) Visual field charting?

Answers

2. (a) Simple partial epilepsy originating in the left uncus in a left hemisphere dominant patient.
   (b) Androgen failure, due to drugs, testicular or pituitary disease.
   (c) This is often psychogenic but is also seen in autonomic disorders and hyperprolactinaemia.
   (d) Drugs, e.g. methyldopa, phenothiazines or reserpine, and hyperprolactinaemia from prolactinoma or in acromegaly.
   (e) The palmomental reflex, like the grasp, pout and suckle reflexes, is a frontal lobe release sign, the presence of which is physiological in patients over the age of 55. Asymmetry is significant and suggests disease in the frontal region.

3. (a) **True**
   (b) **True**
   (c) **True**
   (d) **True**
   (e) **True**

Investigations are required to identify the pituitary lesion, establish any endocrine abnormality and exclude an alternate seizure source. Visual fields should be charted to assess the effects of medical or surgical treatment. A lateral skull radiograph is required in patients with visual failure or a visual field defect, to show the size of the pituitary fossa. The definitive investigation is cranial CT. Angiography is usually required to exclude an aneurysm. Pituitary function tests include serum prolactin, thyroxine, 11-hydroxycorticosteroids and testosterone; dynamic tests are also undertaken, apart from an insulin stress test which is contra-indicated in patients with seizures.

Comment

Serum prolactin was 23 000 units/l (normal <400 units/l). Skull radiography showed an enlarged pituitary fossa and cranial CT showed a large tumour extending out of the pituitary fossa, an appearance confirmed by angiography. The patient was initially treated with bromocriptine; after the tumour had shrunk it was resected by the trans-sphenoidal route.

Further reading

HALL, R., ANDERSON, J., SMART, G. A. and BESSER, M., 'Anterior pituitary', *Fundamentals of Clinical Endocrinology* (1980), Pitman Medical, London, Chapter 1

Case 6.6 Recent memory loss

A 48-year-old woman of low intelligence, who had been unsteady in her walking most of her life, was taken to see her general practitioner by her sister because she had become incontinent of urine. Detailed questioning revealed increasing difficulty in doing the shopping and managing simple household tasks, but no other symptoms of neurological significance. Her son had multiple sclerosis and was confined to a wheelchair. There was no other family history of any neurological disorder. She was a non-smoker and was on no other medication.

On examination she was orientated in time, place and person. On testing memory she was able to register information but could not recall more than two items out of six after 5 min and long-term memory was patchy. She could repeat five digits forwards and four backwards. On testing serial 7s she reached 72 after 30 seconds. Thought content was normal but affect labile. She was unable to explain the true meaning of a proverb. Sense of smell was normal. Visual acuity was J6 in both eyes; the optic discs and pupillary reflexes were normal; upward conjugate gaze was reduced by 50%. She was ataxic in the limbs and on testing gait. Tendon stretch reflexes were brisk and the plantar reflexes extensor. There was a pout reflex, and grasp and palmomental reflexes were present on each side. Neck, skull and hairline were normal.

Questions

1. The following concerning her cognitive functioning may be true or false:
    (a) The findings are compatible with poor academic achievement.
    (b) She has a global dementia.
    (c) Signs suggest patchy hemispheric disease.
    (d) She is depressed.
    (e) She has the Korsakoff psychosis.

Answers

1. (a) **False**
   (b) **False**
   (c) **False**
   (d) **False**
   (e) **True**

Testing cognitive function in patients with poor academic achievement is difficult. This patient's signs suggest recent onset of difficulty with memory, some mild impairment of concentration and attention, and lack of ability to reason. This is less than would be expected in global dementia and more in keeping with the midline or axial dementia seen in the lesions affecting the medial aspect of the temporal lobes or in Korsakoff's psychosis. Hemispheric disease usually causes more spatial or motor signs, e.g. apraxia, and she does not have the disorder of affect seen in a pseudodementia.

Questions

2. Which of the following should be included in the differential diagnosis:

   (a) Hydrocephalus?
   (b) Subfrontal meningioma?
   (c) Glioma of the corpus callosum?
   (d) Alzheimer's disease?
   (e) Alcohol abuse?

3. Which of the following investigations is indicated:

   (a) CSF examination?
   (b) Cranial CT?
   (c) Ventriculography?
   (d) Nerve conduction velocity?
   (e) Measurement of plasma γ-glutamyltransferase (γ-GT) concentration?

Answers

2. (a) **True**
   (b) **True**
   (c) **False**
   (d) **False**
   (e) **True**

Apart from axial dementia, signs suggest supratentorial (primitive reflexes) and infratentorial (failure of upward conjugate gaze, ataxia) disease. The absence of papilloedema would not preclude longstanding hydrocephalus due to aqueduct stenosis or tumour, e.g. meningioma. Gliomas of the corpus callosum usually present with a shorter history and seizures. Alzheimer's disease rarely present with these focal signs. Alcohol abuse is one of the commoner causes of an axial dementia.

3. (a) **True**
   (b) **True**
   (c) **False**
   (d) **False**
   (e) **True**

Hydrocephalus and a tumour should be excluded by cranial CT and the CSF then examined for a pleocytosis which might indicate inflammatory disease. Ventriculography is no longer performed, and nerve conduction studies are not indicated as there is no evidence of a peripheral neuropathy. An elevated serum γ-GT might indicate liver damage in a patient abusing alcohol.

Comment

Cranial CT showed hydrocephalus with enlarged lateral and IIIrd ventricles but normal IVth ventricle – an appearance suggestive of aqueduct stenosis. Cerebral sulci were visible, suggesting that this was chronic. A medium-pressure ventriculoperitoneal shunt was inserted in view of the recent deterioration: although gait improved slightly, there was no overall change in mentation.

Further reading

PICKARD, J. D., 'Adult communicating hydrocephalus', *British Journal of Hospital Medicine* (1982), **29**, 35–44

Exercise 7

Case 7.1 Neurological complications of systemic disease

At the age of 25 years, a previously fit woman was found to have tuberculosis, was treated by thoracoplasty, and later streptomycin, PAS and INH. At the age of 40 she developed swelling of the distal interphalangeal and wrist joints of both hands, attributed to rheumatoid arthritis. Symptoms initially responded to simple analgesics but, 2 years later, she became seropositive and required penicillamine and steroids to control symptoms in the larger joints. At the age of 45 years she was found to be passing 3–4 g protein daily in her urine and was in mild renal failure. Six weeks before admission at the age of 59 years her right thumb became weak in flexion and she was unable to grip. Three weeks later she developed a left wrist drop. Up to 3 years previously she had worked in a paint factory. She smoked 40 cigarettes a day and accompanied her husband to the local working men's club twice a week, where she drank 'Carlsberg Special' lager.

She had signs attributable to her thoracoplasty, including a Horner's syndrome. She was pale with leuconychia; her kidneys were palpable although not irregular. There were changes in the joints compatible with rheumatoid arthritis. On neurological examination she was weak in flexor pollicis longus on the right and brachioradialis and the wrist and finger extensors on the left. There was a small patch of sensory loss on the back of the left thumb.

Questions

1. Which peripheral nerves are likely to be involved:

   (a) Anterior interosseous nerve?
   (b) Posterior interosseous nerve?
   (c) Radial nerve?
   (d) Median nerve?
   (e) Ulnar nerve?

Answers

1. (a) **True**
   (b) **True**
   (c) **False**
   (d) **False**
   (e) **False**

The signs are compatible with an anterior interosseous nerve palsy (weakness in flexor pollicus longus). and a posterior interosseous nerve palsy (weakness in brachioradialis and the wrist and finger extensors). A radial nerve palsy would include weakness in triceps. A median nerve palsy would include weakness in abductor pollicus brevis. The ulnar nerve supplies the long flexors of the medial digits of the hand abductor digiti minimi and the first dorsal interosseous; these muscles are not weak.

Questions

2. Which of these diseases might cause this patient's symptoms:
    (a) Vasculitis?
    (b) Amyloid infiltration?
    (c) A toxic neuropathy?
    (d) Renal failure?
    (e) Alcohol abuse?

Answers

2. (a) **True**
   (b) **False**
   (c) **False**
   (d) **False**
   (e) **False**

There are a number of possible causes. She may have subclinical damage to the peripheral nerves as a result of renal failure, but this alone is unlikely to cause mononeuritis multiplex. She has a long and complicated drug history but toxic neuropathies, like those of uraemia and alcohol abuse, tend to be symmetrical. Isoniazid, which is toxic in slow acetylators, may cause an acute neuropathy in patients not given pyridoxine and she did not receive ethambutol, which causes both an optic and peripheral neuropathy. Penicillamine induces myasthenia which is usually reversible on stopping the drug. Primary amyloid is rare and the congenital form does not present with mononeuritis multiplex. An acquired amyloid neuropathy is often associated with autonomic symptoms and causes mononeuritis multiplex only in the presence of diseases such as myeloma. A vasculitic mononeuritis simplex or multiplex characteristically presents with pain in the distribution of the affected nerve and sudden sensory loss or weakness. Causes include polyarteritis, systemic lupus erythematosis, sarcoid and small vessel disease in diabetes mellitus.

Questions

3. Which of the following investigations would be indicated:

    (a) Nerve conduction studies?
    (b) Nerve biopsy?
    (c) Blood glucose estimation?
    (d) Serum autoantibodies?
    (e) Urinary porphyrin estimation?

4. Which of the following should be used in the management of this patient:

    (a) Administration of steroids?
    (b) Administration of azathioprine?
    (c) Plasmaphaeresis?
    (d) Thymectomy?

Answers

3. (a) **True**
   (b) **True**
   (c) **True**
   (d) **True**
   (e) **True**

Nerve conduction studies and electromyography may be used to localize the lesion. Lesions were found in the anterior and posterior interosseous nerves. There was mild slowing of conduction velocity with evidence of denervation, including positive sharp waves and fibrillation potentials, and a reduced interference pattern on maximal volitional activity compatible with a mild chronic axonal neuropathy, e.g. due to uraemia. A demyelinating neuropathy would be expected to cause slowing of conduction with little evidence of active denervation. Diabetes and other metabolic diseases including porphyria should be excluded. The presence of serum autoantibodies may suggest an underlying collagen vascular disease. A nerve biopsy may show nerve infarcts.

4. (a) **True**
   (b) **True**
   (c) **False**
   (d) **False**

Steroids would be indicated in a patient with collagen vascular disease. Azathioprine is used as an immunosuppressive agent and for its steroid-sparing effect. There is no evidence that plasmaphaeresis or thymectomy are of benefit in these disorders.

Comment

This woman had a mononeuritis multiplex caused by vasculitis secondary to a collagen vascular disease. Nerve and renal biopsy showed evidence of vasculitis. Treatment with steroids and azathioprine improved both renal and neurological function.

Further reading

ADAMS, R. D. and VICTOR, M., 'Diseases of peripheral and cranial nerves', *Principles of Neurology* (1986), McGraw-Hill, New York, Chapter 26

Case 7.2 Abnormal behaviour

A 19-year-old man, a first-year university student, was admitted to a psychiatric hospital from his Hall of Residence because of abnormal behaviour. On admission he was asleep but could be wakened although he remained drowsy and continued to sleep for long periods. On waking he would eat voraciously, requesting extra food between meals. He was seen to masturbate in public and attempted to molest female nursing staff on several occasions. When his parents were contacted they admitted there had been two episodes of similar behaviour when he was 14 and 16 years old.

Questions

1. What is the diagnosis?
2. What investigations are required?
3. What treatment should be given?
4. What is the prognosis?

Answers

1. The Kleine–Levin syndrome.
2. With such a clear-cut history no further investigations are required. Exceptionally, symptoms may be due to a diencephalic tumour and patients should be investigated by cranial CT and EEG during their first attack. Neuroendocrine function is normal.
3. No treatment is known to limit or prevent attacks.
4. The prognosis is good as patients rarely have more than two or three attacks; each attack is self limiting, lasting only a few days or, at most, weeks.

Comment

The Kleine–Levin syndrome is an uncommon syndrome affecting young males and is characterized by periodic hypersomnolence, hyperphagia and, during episodes, evidence of hypersexuality.

Further reading

GARLAND, H., SUMNER, D. and FOURMAN, P., 'The Kleine–Levin syndrome. Some further observations', *Neurology (Minneapolis)* (1965), **15**, 1161

Case 7.3 Deteriorating school work

An 8-year-old girl was taken to her GP by her parents, at the suggestion of her school teacher. In the previous year school performance had deteriorated and learning skills not developed. To the parents she seemed a healthy, attentive, alert and intelligent child. The GP could find no significant abnormality and contacted the school medical officer, who discussed the case with teacher and school friends. They said that at times the girl was vague and slow to answer questions, which had to be repeated, as sometimes there was a delay of some seconds before answering. Neurological examination was unremarkable but for a few seconds she was in a trance, blinking her eyes and unaware of being questioned. Upon recovery she was entirely normal and was unaware of the lapse.

Questions

1. What is the diagnosis?
2. What does this EEG (*Figure 7a*) show?

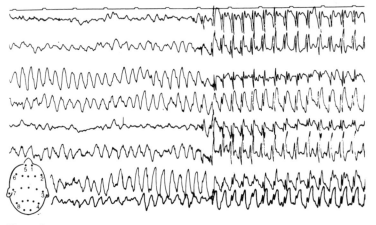

Figure 7a

3. What is the treatment of choice for this condition?

Answers

1. Primary generalized absence epilepsy (petit mal).
2. The EEG (*Figure 7a*) showed 3 Hz spike and wave activity which is characteristic of this type of seizure disorder.
3. Sodium valproate; ethosuximide is second choice.

Comment

Learning difficulties are common in young children and may be difficult to spot and diagnose. Transient lapses of awareness due to epilepsy may become manifest as a general decline in cognitive skills. Children themselves may be unaware of these attacks. Primary generalized absence epilepsy is a dominantly inherited disorder with variable penetrance. A significant percentage of children stop having attacks in their teens but between 30% and 50% will have generalized tonic clonic epilepsy when they reach adulthood.

Further reading

LAIDLAW, J. and RICHENS, A., 'Petit mal', *A Textbook of Epilepsy*, 2nd edition, (1982), Churchill Livingstone, Edinburgh, 51

Case 7.4 Acute dizziness

A 66-year-old man was admitted to hospital having collapsed while gardening. He had been treated for hypertension for 10 years with a β-blocker. Three years previously he had an uncomplicated myocardial infarction. Six months previously he had an episode of dizziness, unsteadiness and slurred speech of sudden onset which lasted a few hours. Six weeks previously he had a further episode when out walking in the street, when he became acutely vertiginous and collapsed to the ground, unable to walk or speak clearly. On the day of admission he again became vertiginous, complained of double vision and collapsed to the ground. He was carried into the house by his family and vomited profusely for half an hour. On admission he was alert and orientated but distressed because any sudden movement rendered him dizzy and caused him to vomit. Blood pressure was 190/110 mmHg. He had a grade II hypertensive retinopathy but there was no other visual abnormality. There was impairment of upward conjugate gaze, and downward conjugate gaze elicited vertical nystagmus. Leftward gaze was partially impaired and, on right horizontal gaze, the right eye abducted fully, but the left eye did not move. The left side of the face was weak. He was unable to sit up because of a truncal ataxia and was ataxic in his left arm. Power was normal, tendon stretch reflexes were brisk and the right plantar reflex extensor. Sensory testing revealed no abnormality.

Questions

1. What is the pathophysiology of these attacks?
2. Where is the lesion anatomically?

By the following day the patient was no longer vomiting and could sit up in bed. He was still unable to walk and objective signs were unchanged. Overnight, however, his condition deteriorated and once more he became vertiginous, speech deteriorated and he developed a complete gaze palsy on leftward gaze and the left side of his face became paralysed.

Questions

3. Why has he deteriorated?
4. What should be the subsequent management?

Answers

1. Vertebrobasilar transient ischaemic attacks.
2. Impairment of vertical conjugate gaze suggests a lesion in the midbrain. He has a gaze palsy to the left and left-sided internuclear ophthalmoplegia which, with the ataxia, would suggest a lesion in the left side of the pons.
3. Progressing thrombosis causing a further area of infarction. This carries a high mortality rate.
4. The patient should undergo cranial CT and examination of the spinal fluid to exclude haemorrhage. Once this is done it would be appropriate to give anticoagulant therapy with intravenous heparin.

Despite treatment his condition deteriorated over the next 48 h. He appeared to be unconscious and was unable to move any limbs. To pain or a vocal stimulus he was able to open his eyes and to command he could look up and down. There was no horizontal movement of either eye, and no movement of either side of the face or bulbar musculature. Tone in the limbs was increased and there appeared to be no voluntary movement on either side. Tendon stretch reflexes were all brisk and the plantar reflexes were extensor.

Question

5. What is the explanation of this combination of signs?

Answer

5. This is the 'locked-in' syndrome.

Comment

In the 'locked-in' syndrome there is damage below the level of the rostral part of the third nerve nucleus, sparing vertical eye movement and the reticular activating system, thus allowing a conscious patient to communicate by eye movement. Lesions are usually ischaemic in origin and there is a very poor prognosis for further recovery.

Further reading

PLUM, F. and POSNER, J. B., 'Locked-in syndrome', *The Diagnosis of Stupor and Coma*, 3rd edition (1980), F. A. Davis Co., Philadelphia, 9

Case 7.5 Painful blindness

A 17-year-old girl presented with a 3-day history of pain and blurred vision in the right eye, progressing to almost complete blindness. There was no previous history. Examination revealed a large central scotoma most marked to red light; the visual acuity was less than 6/60 in the right eye but normal on the left. The optic fundi were normal and there was no pupillary response to light in the right eye but normal constriction of both pupils to light in the left eye.

Questions

1. The following statements concerning this patient's visual failure may be true or false:

    (a) Painful visual loss suggests ophthalmoplegic migraine.
    (b) Acute visual loss indicates central retinal vein thrombosis.
    (c) The findings suggest a right optic neuropathy,
    (d) Failure of pupillary light reflexes suggest a partial IIIrd nerve lesion.
    (e) Visual evoked responses would be expected to be normal.

Answers

1. (a) **False**
   (b) **False**
   (c) **True**
   (d) **False**
   (e) **False**

The history and clinical findings, including the failure of either pupil to constrict in response to light shone in the right eye, suggest an afferent pupillary defect. This occurs in an optic neuropathy when torsion of the swollen nerve causes pain. This would be confirmed by a delayed VEP. A normal optic fundus excludes a central retinal artery or vein thrombosis in which there is a haemorrhagic retinopathy. Ophthalmoplegic migraine causes IIIrd, IVth and VIth nerve palsy without any alteration in visual acuity.

Treatment was instituted and vision returned to normal within 6 weeks. At the age of 21 years, during her first pregnancy, she developed urgency and frequency of micturition, and a sensation of numbness extending from the feet to the mid-trunk. The latter resolved spontaneously over 6 weeks but urgency and frequency of micturition persisted.

At the age of 25 years, 3 days after having given birth to a boy, she was admitted to hospital with vertigo, unsteadiness and double vision of acute onset. A maternal aunt was known to have had episodes of double vision in her early 20s and at the age of 25 years was wheelchair-bound due to a condition which the patient described as neuritis.

Questions

2. The following statements about the symptoms and their onset may be true or false:

   (a) The onset suggests a diagnosis of benign positional vertigo.
   (b) Brain-stem symptoms evolving in this way in a young woman suggest a pontine glioma.
   (c) The temporal pattern suggests a demyelinating disorder.
   (d) The relationship between the onset of symptoms and delivery of the child is coincidental.
   (e) Evoked response studies might help to confirm the diagnosis.

142

Answers

2. (a) **False**
   (b) **False**
   (c) **True**
   (d) **True**
   (e) **True**

A history of relapsing and remitting neurological signs affecting several different sites within the neuraxis would suggest demyelinating disease. There is an increased risk of relapse during pregnancy. Evoked response studies may be used to demonstrate sites of subclinical disease within the neuraxis but are not in themselves diagnostic of multiple sclerosis. Benign positional vertigo would not explain cerebellar signs and a pontine glioma would not be preceded by these visual symptoms.

On examination, uncorrected visual acuity on the left was J1 and on the right J4. The right optic disc was pale. Pupillary reflexes were present. There was horizontal phasic nystagmus on gaze to the right; on gaze left the right eye failed to adduct and the left eye showed coarse nystagmus. There was upbeat nystagmus on upward vertical conjugate gaze. She was ataxic when sitting and was titubating. She was unable to stand or walk unsupported. She had an intention tremor of both arms and the legs were clumsy. She had a cerebellar dysarthria. Power was normal but the tendon stretch reflexes were pathologically brisk with a brisk jaw jerk. Abdominal reflexes were absent and plantar reflexes extensor. Visual evoked responses were delayed from the right eye. Brain-stem evoked responses were abnormal bilaterally. CSF examination revealed fluid under normal pressure, containing 15 lymphocytes/μl and 0.6 g/l protein, of which 35% was IgG and oligoclonal bands were present.

Questions

3. The following concerning management and prognosis may be true or false:

   (a) Recent pregnancy is a contra-indication to the use of steroids.

   (b) Risks of further acute episodes with future pregnancies are slight.

   (c) The presence of a similar illness in another family member is unlikely to influence prognosis.

144

Answers

3. (a) **False**
   (b) **False**
   (c) **False**

Steroids have been shown to shorten the length of relapse in patients with retrobulbar neuritis and are widely used to treat relapses in patients with multiple sclerosis. Recent pregnancy is not a contra-indication to their use. Patients with multiple sclerosis are recognized to have increased risk of exacerbation during pregnancy and the first 3 months of the puerperium. There is a significant risk (7–10-fold) that other members of the family may develop the disease and therefore the presence of the disease in an aunt is not merely coincidental.

Comment

Multiple sclerosis is not infrequently seen in more than one member of a family. Young patients with disease involving the cerebellar connections have a poor prognosis in functional terms.

Further reading

McAlpine's Multiple Sclerosis (1985) (ed. Matthews, W. B.), Churchill Livingstone, Edinburgh

Case 7.6 Sudden falls

An 18-year-old boy suffered a minor injury at his local youth club. He had been playing table tennis when he fell and caught the side of his head against the edge of the table. He sustained a small laceration above the right eye, requiring two stitches, but there were no other injuries. The casualty officer was concerned about the nature of the fall and asked the neurological registrar to see the patient.

On detailed questioning it emerged that the boy had collapsed rather than fallen. He had made a winning backhand stroke and cried out. He claimed that his legs gave way beneath him and he fell unable to protect himself: as a result of this his head hit the edge of the table. He was not rendered unconscious and was able to get up immediately. He admitted a number of similar falls, the first at the age of 15 years when standing at his first Communion, when his legs 'felt like jelly' and he fell on to his knees. Similar episodes occurred on a number of subsequent occasions – all times of intense emotion. One episode he remembered very vividly was when a young cousin had come up to him at a party and said 'Let me hold your hand so you won't fall': this had produced the most dramatic fall of them all. Previously there had never been any injury.

Questions

1. What is the cause of this syndrome?
2. What other direct questions should be asked?
3. What is the most likely underlying diagnosis?
4. What investigations are indicated?
5. What treatment is indicated?
6. What is the prognosis?

Answers

1. A fall precipitated by emotion is cataplexy.
2. (a) Are there episodes of unprovoked, irresistible sleep from which he can be woken by touch?
   (b) Are there nightmares or hallucinations?
   (c) Are there episodes of paralysis?
3. Narcolepsy triad or tetrad.
4. No investigations are indicated. Very occasionally excessive sleepiness may be due to respiratory disease or intracranial tumour, or may follow head injury.
5. Clomipramine may reduce the number of cataplectic attacks and methylphenidate usually prevents narcolepsy.
6. The condition is not life threatening in itself. Attacks continue throughout life.

Comment

The narcolepsy tetrad consists of narcolepsy, cataplexy, hypnogogic (falling asleep) or hypnopompic (waking) hallucinations and sleep paralysis. Cataplexy may be provoked by any emotional stimulus and may vary in severity from a feeling of weakness to a fall. Injury is uncommon.

Further reading

PARKS, J. D., 'Narcolepsy and cataplexy', *Quarterly Journal of Medicine* (1974). **43**, 525

Exercise 8

Case 8.1 A painful shaking limb

A 55-year-old right-handed housewife presented with a 6-month history of pain and stiffness in the right arm, which had been resistant to simple analgesics. Two weeks previously she developed a constant tremor in the right arm which became most noticeable when she was sitting at home in the evenings. It was made worse by emotional stress and caused difficulty with household tasks such as knitting and sewing. Writing had become illegible and she had notified her bank of a change in signature. A maternal aunt had a tremor late in life but the patient's own parents were alive and well in their late 70s. She was on no medication and there was no past medical history.

Questions

1. The following statements concerning the history may be true or false:
   (a) Tremor in the right arm suggests a left cerebellar hemisphere lesion.
   (b) Pain and stiffness may be due to frozen shoulder.
   (c) Parkinson's disease would not cause unilateral symptoms.
   (d) Family history of tremor may be relevant.
   (e) Symptoms may be due to thyrotoxicosis.

148

Answers

1. (a) **False**
   (b) **True**
   (c) **False**
   (d) **True**
   (e) **False**

She has a resting tremor associated with stiffness in the same limb. Benign familial and metabolic tremors (e.g. thyrotoxicosis) are usually bilateral and appear on action. Cerebellar tremors are ipsilateral. Parkinson's disease is often initially unilateral and may result in a frozen shoulder which may cause pain and additional stiffness in the affected limb.

Examination revealed an expressionless face, generalized stiffness, poverty of movement and a compound resting tremor of the right arm. She had a dorsal kyphosis and loss of associated movements in the right arm when walking. There was a glabellar tap. In both arms increased tone was 'cogwheel' in type. Power was normal. Tendon stretch reflexes were physiological.

Questions

2. The following concerning management may be true or false:

   (a) A right stereotactic thalamotomy would reduce stiffness.
   (b) The tremor would be reduced by anticholinergic drugs.
   (c) Start of treatment should be deferred.
   (d) Levodopa would produce consideral functional improvement.
   (e) Administration of selegeline is indicated.

Answers

2. (a) **False**
   (b) **True**
   (c) **True**
   (d) **True**
   (e) **False**

It is now generally accepted that it is right to defer treatment for Parkinson's disease until functional activity is impaired. The treatment of choice is levodopa in combination with a peripheral decarboxylase inhibitor for bradykinesia and rigidity, although there is some evidence that anticholinergic drugs may be better in reducing tremor. Selegeline (an MAO-B inhibitor) may be an adjunct to dopaminergic treatment but probably has little action on its own. Patients with a severe tremor which is resistant to medical treatment should be considered for contralateral thalamotomy, but this would not affect the other symptoms.

She was treated with a combination of levodopa (750 mg) and a dopa-decarboxylase inhibitor (75 mg) daily. Her disease remained well controlled for 6 years but then she developed periods of immobility alternating with involuntary movements. The latter consisted of facial and limb dyskinesias which stopped her sitting still and appeared within 30 min of taking her tablets.

Questions

3. The following statements may be true or false:

    (a) The original diagnosis was incorrect.
    (b) These fluctuations do not occur with anticholinergic drugs alone.
    (c) Symptoms are due to levodopa.
    (d) Thalamotomy will relieve the dyskinesia.
    (e) The recent change is the natural history of the disease.

Answers

3. (a) **False**
   (b) **True**
   (c) **True**
   (d) **False**
   (e) **False**

She now has 'beginning-of-dose dyskinesia'. This occurs in patients with Parkinson's disease after long periods of treatment with levodopa. The original diagnosis is not in doubt and this is drug effect, rather than being part of the natural course of the disease. These dyskinesias do not occur in patients treated with anticholinergic drugs and do not respond to thalamotomy.

Comment

It is important to categorize the type of dyskinesia. Beginning-of-dose, peak dose and end-of-dose dyskinesias are seen in patients who have received levodopa for between 3 and 10 years. They may reflect supersensitivity of the dopamine receptor or altered amino-acid absorption from the bowel. Smaller doses of levodopa given more frequently may reduce peak and end-of-dose dyskinesias. Patients tolerate beginning-of-dose dyskinesias better if given larger doses of levodopa less frequently.

Further reading

MARSDEN, C. D., PARKES, J. D. and QUINN, N., 'Fluctuations of disability in Parkinson's disease – clinical aspects', (eds Marsden, C. D. and Fahn, S.), *Movement Disorders, Neurology 2* (1982), Butterworths International Medical Reviews, Chapter 7

Case 8.2 Pain in the chest

A 60-year-old lady was admitted to hospital with a rapidly evolving spastic paraparesis. She had been attending a chiropractor for 5 years because of pain between the shoulder blades and a tight band-like sensation around the chest. For 12 months she had had urgency and frequency of micturition and had been incontinent on several occasions, all of which she had ascribed to a vaginal prolapse. Her paraparesis had evolved over 5 days and the night before admission she developed retention of urine.

On examination her skin was normal. She was tender over D4. She had a spastic paraparesis with a motor level above the umbilicus but below the T1 innervated muscles. There was a symmetrical sensory level at D10 with sacral sparing. Tendon stretch reflexes were brisk in the lower limbs and normal in the upper limbs. There was sustained clonus at each ankle and both plantar reflexes were extensor.

Questions

1. The following concerning the history and signs may be true or false:

   (a) Interscapular pain suggests a disc prolapse.
   (b) The length of the history suggests a secondary tumour deposit.
   (c) Sacral sparing suggests a lesion in the thoracic spinal cord.
   (d) A sensory level at D10 is compatible with a lesion at the level of the 6th dorsal vertebral body.
   (e) They are compatible with cervical spondylosis.

2. The following concerning management may be true or false:

   (a) Lumbar spine radiographs should be obtained.
   (b) CSF examination is indicated.
   (c) Dorsal spine transverse CT is the investigation of choice.
   (d) Myelography is indicated.

Answers

1. (a) **True**
   (b) **False**
   (c) **True**
   (d) **True**
   (e) **False**

A history of interscapular and radicular pain and an evolving paraparesis suggest a longstanding structural lesion, not a secondary deposit, lying in the dorsal spinal canal. Differential diagnosis includes neurofibroma or meningioma, prolapsed dorsal disc or congenital abnormality associated with spinal dysraphism. Sacral sparing suggests a lesion in the spinal cord. This clinically appears to be above D10.

2. (a) **False**
   (b) **False**
   (c) **True**
   (d) **True**

Radiological investigation will indicate the site and possible pathology of the lesion. Plain radiographs of the dorsal and cervical spine and myelography with CT demonstrate intra- and extra-axial tumour. CSF should not be examined alone. Myelography should be undertaken only if facilities exist to decompress the lesion as a spinal pressure cone may cause further neurological deterioration.

Comment

No underlying primary tumour was found. Radiography of the dorsal spine showed scalloping of the pedicle and erosion of the posterior aspect of the vertebral body at D4. There was complete obstruction to contrast material on myelography by an extramedullary tumour at D4 with the spinal cord displaced posteriorly. CSF was xanthochromic with a protein content of 5 g/l. No cells were seen. An extramedullary intradural meningioma was resected and the patient made a good recovery with a residual mild spastic paraparesis.

Further reading

WALTON, J. N., 'Spinal tumours', *Brain's Diseases of the Nervous System*, 9th edition (1986), Churchill Livingstone, Edinburgh, 401

Case 8.3 A slater with a headache

A 22-year-old right-handed slater was admitted with a 5-week history of headache, nausea and malaise sufficient to keep him off work. He had been pyrexial for 3 weeks and when he developed a stiff neck and became confused he was admitted to hospital.

On examination he was drowsy and confused when roused. Temperature was 39°C; he was photophobic with neck stiffness and Kernig's sign was present. Blood pressure was 140/85 mmHg; heart rate 120/min. Small lymph nodes were palpable in both axillae. The chest was dull to percussion, with reduced vocal fremitus at the right base and scattered rhonchi throughout. The optic discs were pink but there were no retinal haemorrhages.

Questions

1. What would be the significance of the following findings in this patient:

    (a) General malaise and localizing pulmonary signs?
    (b) Neck stiffness and photophobia?
    (c) Small white glistening bodies away from the optic nerve head on retinal examination?
    (d) Elevated CSF protein?
    (e) Dilated ventricular system on cranial CT?

2. Which of the following should be included in the differential diagnosis:

    (a) Cryptococcosis?
    (b) Ruptured mycotic aneurysm?
    (c) AIDS?
    (d) Tuberculosis?
    (e) Viral meningitis?

Answers

1. The symptoms and signs suggest a generalized infective illness with involvement of the pulmonary and nervous systems.

    (a) Pleural effusion with probable underlying consolidation.
    (b) Meningitis.
    (c) Choroidal tubercles which are diagnostic of tuberculosis.
    (d) This is a non-specific finding which indicates either damage to the blood–brain barrier, e.g. in infection or certain tumours, or synthesis of one of the component proteins, e.g. IgG within the neuraxis. In this context the former is likely.
    (e) Hydrocephalus may result from a high protein level or, more probably, obstruction to the CSF drainage pathways by inflammatory exudate.

2. (a) **True**
    (b) **False**
    (c) **True**
    (d) **True**
    (e) **True**

The differential diagnosis of a subacute meningitis includes tuberculosis, cryptococcosis and other opportunistic infections including toxoplasmosis in patients with an immune deficiency syndrome. Cryptococcosis, carried by birds, is an occupational disease of slaters, although rare: CSF cryptococcal antibody and antigen levels should be measured. A ruptured mycotic aneurysm presents as an intracranial haematoma with subarachnoid haemorrhage.

He had proteinuria with polymorphs and lymphocytes in the urine; no organisms were seen. Haemoglobin was 12 g/dl, white cell count 17 000 with a relative lymphocytosis. ESR 68 mm/h. Chest radiography showed scattered lesions throughout the lung fields and there was a small right basal pulmonary effusion. The latter contained elevated protein, low glucose and polymorphs. Cranial CT was normal. CSF opening pressure was 210 mm. There were 210 white cells/μl, 90% lymphocytes, protein was 3.2 g/l and glucose 1.2 mmol/l (blood glucose 7.3 mmol/l). Acid-fast rod-shaped organisms were seen.

Treatment was given and he slowly improved. On discharge 4 weeks later CSF protein was 0.8 g/l and there were 10 lymphocytes/μl.

Eighteen months after the original illness the patient developed a mild but slowly progressive weakness of both legs. On examination he had a spastic paraparesis, brisk tendon stretch reflexes and a sensory level at D8.

Questions

3. (a) What structure is involved to cause the present weakness?
   (b) Name two possible mechanisms in relation to his previous illness.
   (c) What investigations are indicated?
   (d) What is the prognosis for recovery?

Answers

3. (a) Spinal cord.
   (b) (i) Pott's disease of the spine with spinal cord compression due to a cold abscess or vertebral collapse.
   (ii) Arachnoiditis.
   (c) Plain radiography of the dorsal spine and, if normal, myelography with CSF examination.
   (d) Pott's disease of the spine would require immobilization and further antituberculous treatment: it carries a relatively good prognosis for recovery. Arachnoiditis may respond to steroids but prognosis for recovery is not good.

Plain radiographs were normal. Lumbar myelography showed irregularities throughout the lumbar and lower dorsal subarachnoid space with a complete obstruction to contrast at D6. Cervical myelography showed a normal subarachnoid space down to C8 but similar irregular filling defects below this level. This appearance was thought to indicate arachnoiditis. CSF opening pressure was 80 mmHg. The CSF was yellow and contained protein 6.1 g/l and glucose 3.4 mmol/l (blood glucose 4.4 mmol/l).

Comment

In basal or spinal arachnoiditis following tuberculosis the inflammatory process ultimately compromises the blood supply to the spinal cord. Ischaemia and infarction may progress over months or years, causing cranial nerve palsies, radiculopathies and a myelopathy. Treatment with steroids is not satisfactory and the prognosis for recovery is poor.

Further reading

ASHWORTH, B. and SAUNDERS, M., 'Infection and infestations', *Management of Neurological Disorders*, 2nd edition (1985), Butterworths, London, Chapter 19

Case 8.4 Headache and a weak arm

A 45-year-old White Caucasian woman presented with a 4-week history of headache and weakness in the left arm. Headaches were frontal and, as time passed, became more intense and continued by day and night. She lost her appetite 1 week before admission and on 3 different days vomited after waking in the morning with a headache. Her left arm had become clumsy and she had increasing difficulty in manipulating small objects. In the previous year she had lost 11 kg in weight. She had a cough, twice with blood-stained sputum.

On examination she looked ill. She had finger clubbing. Optic fundi and eye movements were normal. There was a mild degree of left lower facial weakness and the outstretched left arm tended to drift downwards. Fine finger movements were impaired on the left. Tendon stretch reflexes were brisker on the left. Legs were normal other than an extensor plantar reflex on the left. There were no sensory abnormalities.

Questions

1. The following interpretations of her symptoms and signs may be true or false:

   (a) There is a lesion in the left cerebellar hemisphere.
   (b) There is a lesion in the right parietal lobe.
   (c) There is no evidence of raised intracranial pressure.
   (d) Tuberculosis is the most likely diagnosis.

Answers

1. (a) **False**
   (b) **True**
   (c) **False**
   (d) **False**

Signs indicate a lesion in the right frontoparietal region (contralateral pyramidal signs), not the cerebellum. The history is suggestive of raised intracranial pressure; papilloedema need not be present as it takes time to develop clinically. Signs suggest a rapidly expanding mass lesion and the most likely diagnosis is a bronchogenic tumour with cerebral secondaries.

ESR was 56 mm/h. Chest radiography showed an opacity in the right apex. Cranial CT confirmed the presence of an enhancing lesion in the right frontal region with considerable surrounding oedema. There were malignant squamous cells on sputum cytology. Neurological signs improved with administration of corticosteroids. She died 3 months later and at autopsy was found to have an squamous cell tumour with extensive metastasis including a large necrotic tumour in the right frontal lobe.

Comment

Rapidly expanding intracranial lesions in adults frequently turn out to be metastases. Patients require investigation including chest radiography, abdominal ultrasound and sputum and urine cytology. Quality of life may be improved when peritumoral oedema is reduced by steroids or radiotherapy but only rarely is it justified to remove the tumour surgically.

Further reading

JENNETT, B. and GALBRAITH, S., 'Intranial tumours'. *An Introduction to Neurosurgery*, 4th edition (1983), Heinemann, London, Chapter 8

Case 8.5 A painful eye

A 52-year-old man had a 6-week history of pain in the right eye. He was hypertensive and had maturity-onset diabetes. His mother had had multiple sclerosis and died 8 years previously of bronchopneumonia.

On examination blood pressure was 180/105 mmHg. He had a quiet systolic bruit over the left carotid artery. Sense of smell was preserved. Visual acuity was J2 in both eyes. Visual fields were full to confrontation. The right pupil was dilated with no direct pupillary light reflex, although the left constricted. On testing, the left eye constricted directly but there was no response on the right. There was a full range of eye movement. The lower cranial nerves were normal.

Questions

1. What two anatomical structures are involved?
2. What is the probable pathology?
3. What is the investigation of choice?

Answers

1. (a) Parasympathetic pupilloconstrictor fibres of the oculomotor nerve.
   (b) Ophthalmic division of the trigeminal nerve.
2. Posterior communicating artery aneurysm.
3. Carotid angiography.

Angiography demonstrated a posterior communicating artery aneurysm which was clipped surgically.

Comment

The signs are those of an efferent pupillary defect. Pupilloconstrictor fibres and those to levator palpabrae superiores lie around the outside of the IIIrd nerve and receive blood supply from the meninges. Compressive lesions cause trigeminal pain (the dura is innervated by the ophthalmic division), pupillary dilatation and ptosis, whereas occlusive arterial lesions cause a painless ophthalmoplegia.

Further reading

SPEZTLER, R. F. and ZABRAMSKI, J. M. 'Surgery of intracranial aneurysms', (eds Barnett, H. J. M., Mohr, J. P., Stein, B. M. and Yatsu, F. M.), *Stroke, Pathophysiology Diagnosis and Management* (1986), Churchill Livingstone, Edinburgh, Chapter 55

Case 8.6 Weakness and a rash

A woman aged 56 years, previously in good health, went on holiday to the south of France. She acquired a sun tan but was surprised by how red her face and hands had become. This persisted longer than expected and during the winter she lost 15 kg and had episodes of abdominal pain. When spring cleaning the following year she was unable to clean the tops of the windows. Over the next 3 weeks she had increasing discomfort in her legs and had difficulty in climbing stairs. She had never smoked. Her husband was an electrician in a shipyard.

On examination she was thin. Blood pressure was 110/60 mmHg and there was a quiet systolic murmur at the left sternal edge. Limb girdle muscles were tender on palpation. There was mild weakness in neck flexion and extension and a more marked weakness proximally in the limbs. Tendon stretch reflexes were brisk; plantar reflexes were flexor. There were no sensory abnormalities. Skin was normal.

Questions

1. The following may be true or false:

   (a) The persisting sun tan is unlikely to be relevant.
   (b) Symptoms suggest an underlying malignant tumour.
   (c) She has a peripheral neuropathy.
   (d) Hypercalcaemia explains the weakness and hyper-reflexia.
   (e) The length of the history is incompatible with polymyositis.

2. The following would be expected to be abnormal:

   (a) Serum creatine kinase activity.
   (b) Nerve conduction velocity.
   (c) Serum myoglobin.
   (d) Thyroid function tests.
   (e) Liver biopsy.

3. The following would be expected on electromyography:

   (a) Bizarre high-frequency discharges.
   (b) Impaired recruitment on maximal voluntary contraction.
   (c) Increased insertional activity.
   (d) An excess of polyphasic potentials.
   (e) A decremental response to repetitive stimulation.

164

Answers

1. (a) **False**
   (b) **True**
   (c) **False**
   (d) **True**
   (e) **False**

The neurological signs suggest a myopathy, which could be secondary to hypercalcaemia in a patient with hyper-reflexia. Patients with dermatomyositis (Type B polymyositis) have a mean time to presentation of 8 months and often the illness begins with a violaceous photosensitive rash. Some patients (mainly elderly males) have been shown to have an increased incidence of malignant disease (Type C polymyositis). It would be important to investigate the history of weight loss and abdominal pain, if only to exclude peptic ulceration before starting treatment.

2. (a) **True**
   (b) **False**
   (c) **True**
   (d) **False**
   (e) **False**

Patients with muscle breakdown have elevated serum creatine kinase and myoglobin activity. There is a rare association between polymyositis and other forms of autoimmune disease but usually thyroid function tests would be normal. Nerve conduction studies (but not EMG) would be normal. Liver histology might be abnormal in patients with vasculitis.

3. (a) **True**
   (b) **False**
   (c) **True**
   (d) **True**
   (e) **False**

Electromyographic changes seen in inflammatory muscle disease include increased insertional activity with fibrillation potentials, positive sharp waves and bizarre high-frequency discharges at 150 Hz which gradually decrease in frequency and amplitude. These are also seen in myotonia. Polyphasic potentials suggest a myopathy. Reduced interference pattern suggests abnormal innervation to muscle, i.e. a neuropathy. A decremental response is seen in myasthenia gravis.

Questions

4. The following histopathological abnormalities might be seen in affected muscle:

   (a) Centrally placed nuclei.
   (b) Fibre-type grouping.
   (c) Abnormal mitochondrial clumps around the edge of the muscle cell.
   (d) An inflammatory exudate.
   (e) Degenerating muscle fibre.

5. The following forms of treatment are indicated:

   (a) Oral corticosteroids.
   (b) Thymectomy.
   (c) Plasmaphaeresis.
   (d) Oral non-steroidal anti-inflammatory drugs.

Answers

4. (a) **True**
   (b) **False**
   (c) **False**
   (d) **True**
   (e) **True**

An infiltrate of mononuclear cells, lymphocytes, histiocytes and plasma cells is seen throughout. Sarcoplasm is eosinophilic with degeneration and phagocytosis of muscle fibres. Small angulated basophilic fibres with centrally placed nuclei indicate regeneration. Denervated muscle undergoing reinnervation shows fibre-type grouping. Abnormal clumps of mitochondria are seen in mitochondrial myopathies.

5. (a) **True**
   (b) **False**
   (c) **False**
   (d) **False**

There are no controlled trials of treatment in polymyositis but patients usually respond to steroids with or without immunosuppression. Some patients benefit from plasmaphaeresis or thymectomy, but these are not accepted treatments. There is no place for NSAIDS.

Comment

Serum creatine kinase activity was 3800 units/l. EMG findings confirmed an underlying inflammatory myopathy. The muscle showed a heavy cellular infiltrate, degenerating fibres, phagocytosis and a few small angulated fibres. She was treated with steroids and azathioprine. A crush fracture at D8 was treated with calcium supplements and oestrogens. No underlying malignant disease was found.

Further reading

HUDGSON, P. and WALTON, J. N., 'Polymyositis and other inflammatory disorders', (eds Vinken, P. J., Bruyn, G. W. and Ringel, S. P.), *Handbook of Clinical Neurology, Vol 41* (1979), North Holland Publishing Co, Amsterdam, Chapter 3

Exercise 9

Case 9.1 Blindness after a road accident

A 45-year-old man was a front-seat passenger in a car which collided with a lamp post. He was not wearing a seat belt and was thrown through the windscreen, sustaining a mild concussional head injury, extensive lacerations over the forehead and right periorbital bruising. Fractures of his right radius and left tibia were treated conservatively. There were no focal neurological signs, but over the next 10 days vision in his right eye gradually deteriorated and, as the periorbital bruising settled, he was noted to have conjunctival injection. Two weeks after the accident he complained of double vision on left and right gaze.

On examination it was noted that the eye was prominent. Acuity in the right eye was reduced to counting fingers, but was normal (J1) on the left. He had a right-sided pulsatile reducible axial proptosis with a bruit over the eye. Eye movements in the right were restricted in all directions of gaze.

Questions

1. What is the most likely diagnosis?
2. What is the prognosis?
3. What investigation and treatment should be undertaken?

Answers

1. Traumatic caroticocavernous fistula.
2. Untreated, the eye would continue to proptose and vision would be lost completely.
3. Carotid angiography followed by surgical closure.

Comment

Traumatic rupture of the carotid artery into the cavernous sinus is rare, but may follow minor injury.

Further reading

JENNETT, B. and TEASDALE, G., 'Caroticocavernous fistula', *Management of Head Injuries* (1981), F. A. Davis Co., Philadelphia, 279

Case 9.2 An unresponsive patient

A 25-year-old woman was admitted as an emergency, having been found at home in an unresponsive state. For 5 years she had been seen by psychiatrists for a variety of symptoms. These included episodes of paranoia for which, 2 years previously, she had been treated with phenothiazines. Her most recent delusion had been 6 months previously. Her husband said that she had been strange for about 4 weeks. She had complained that the neighbours were talking about her and she accused her husband of having an affair. Symptoms had become increasingly florid and she had been wandering around the house talking to herself. Her husband left for work at 8.00 a.m. on the day of admission with his wife apparently asleep in bed; when he returned at lunch time he was unable to communicate with her.

On admission she appeared unresponsive and lay quietly as if asleep, with her eyes closed. To vigorous stimulation her eyes opened but she would neither speak nor obey commands. There were spontaneous rolling eye movements with an intact menace response. The pupils were equal and reactive and the corneal responses on each side were normal. In all limbs there was resistance to passive movement and each withdrew to a painful stimulus. The tendon stretch reflexes were normal. Plantar reflexes were flexor. When either arm was lifted into the air it tended to remain in that position.

Questions

1. What is the probable diagnosis?
2. What is the differential diagnosis?
3. What is the explanation of the positive menace response?
4. Why do the arms remain in any position in which they are placed?
5. What investigation might be required to confirm the diagnosis?

Answers

1. Catatonic schizophrenia with catatonic stupor.
2. Other causes of stupor including depressive stupor, hysterical stupor and organic stupor due to CNS disease.
3. The positive menace response indicates a degree of alertness and intact connections between visual cortex and retina. A positive menace response in a stuporose patient is strongly suggestive of a psychiatric disturbance.
4. This is flexibilitas cerea, a manifestation of catatonia.
5. The most helpful investigation is the EEG. In psychiatric stupor it is normal, whereas in organic CNS stupor there is a diffuse abnormality.

Comment

Psychogenic unresponsiveness must be distinguished from organic stupor. The former may respond dramatically to electro-convulsive therapy, which would be inappropriate in the latter.

Further reading

PLUM, F. and POSNER, J. B., 'Catatonia', *The Diagnosis of Stupor and Coma* (1980), F. A. Davies Co., Philadelphia, 308

Case 9.3 Slow motor development

A 3-year-old boy was referred for assessment of walking difficulty. He was the second son of parents in their mid-20s whose first son, now aged 7 years, had a normal childhood. The patient was delivered normally after a full-term normal pregnancy. Initial assessments and milestones had been normal but whereas his brother had stood at the age of 11 months and taken his first steps at 13 months, this child had not been able to stand until the age of 2 years and, although walking at the age of 3 years, was slow and clumsy. He had fallen on many occasions and had never been able to run. Shortly before his assessment, his parents noted he was tending to pull himself up from the ground using furniture and on one occasion appeared to push himself upright by resting his hands on his knees. There was no known family history of any neurological disorder, but his mother had been adopted. The patient had measles at the age of 2 years without any sequelae. Examination revealed a bright, alert little boy. There was marked wasting of the buttocks and thigh muscles with apparently bulky muscles in the calves and anterior tibial compartments. Shoulder girdles showed similar although less evident wasting and the forearms were normal. There was weakness of the shoulder girdle muscles, most marked in serratus anterior, the pectorals and biceps. In the lower limbs there was gross weakness of iliopsoas, quadriceps and the glutei. The facial and trunk muscles appeared relatively strong but the child had difficulty sitting up unaided and when asked to stand from the lying position he used his arms to climb up his own legs. His posture was abnormal with a lumbar lordosis and he walked with a waddling gait. Tendon stretch reflexes were reduced in all four limbs apart from the ankle jerks. No contractures were noted and there were no sensory signs.

Questions

1. The following statements may be true or false:

   (a) The probable diagnosis is facioscapulohumeral dystrophy.
   (b) The age of onset suggests Duchenne muscular dystrophy.
   (c) Serum creatine kinase activity would be normal.
   (d) Histopathological examination of the muscles would show an inflammatory infiltrate.
   (e) One in four children of this marriage will be affected.

Answers

1. (a) **False**
   (b) **True**
   (c) **False**
   (d) **False**
   (e) **True**

The distribution of the weakness and the presence of pseudo-hypertrophy of the calf muscles would suggest the diagnosis is Duchenne muscular dystrophy, not facioscapulohumeral dystrophy: the latter would tend to present much later in life. Investigations expected to confirm muscle breakdown include elevated serum creatine kinase activity, although this falls when the disease burns itself out and little muscle is available for breakdown. Electrophysiological studies help to discriminate between muscular dystrophy and spinal muscular atrophy, and muscle biopsy would be expected to show evidence of fibre atrophy and fibrosis. The disorder is sex linked, with the male affected and the female as the carrier. One child in four of this marriage is likely to suffer from the disease and one in two of any daughters will be carriers.

Comment

Duchenne muscular dystrophy affects young boys and progresses relentlessly to death usually before the age of 20. It is now possible by amniocentesis to determine whether an infant is affected before birth, and to offer termination of an affected pregnancy.

Further reading

WALTON, J. N. and GARDNER-MEDWIN, D., 'Progressive muscular dystrophy and the myotonic disorders', (ed. Walton, J. N.), *Disorders of Voluntary Muscles*, 4th edition, (1981), Churchill Livingstone, Edinburgh, Chapter 14

Case 9.4 A paralysed arm

A man of 19 years was travelling to work on his motorbike and wearing a crash helmet. It was a wet day and he skidded on leaves, landing on his left side and forcibly abducting his left arm. On admission to hospital he was found to have a paralysed left arm and fractured right femur which required internal fixation. When examined by a neurologist 3 weeks later the following left-sided abnormalities were noted: there was ptosis with a small pupil and absence of sweating on the face; the hand was dry and there was wasting of all muscle groups; power was reduced in serratus anterior and rhomboids. He was able to initiate abduction of the shoulder and flexion at the elbow using both biceps and brachioradialis. Extension of the elbow was impaired and there was no movement in the wrists or finger extensors or flexors or the intrinsic muscles of the hand. Biceps and brachioradialis reflexes were retained, although other reflexes in the arm were absent. Sensory testing revealed loss to all modalities in the hand and medial aspect of the arm as far as the axilla.

Questions

1. Which of the following structures is involved:

    (a) Spinal cord?
    (b) Nerve roots?
    (c) Brachial plexus?
    (d) Peripheral nerve?

2. What is the mechanism of this damage?

3. The following may be true or false concerning abnormalities found on investigation:

    (a) Preservation of the weal and flare response on testing the axon reflex.
    (b) Preserved sensory nerve action potentials.
    (c) Active denervation in the small muscles of the hand.
    (d) Normal motor conduction velocities.
    (e) Preservation of the digit II 'F' waves.

Answers

1. (a) **False**
   (b) **True**
   (c) **True**
   (d) **False**

There is evidence of lower motor neurone involvement; the Horner's syndrome suggests that the lesion involves the T1 root as well as the brachial plexus.

2. Two possible mechanisms are involved: first, neurapraxia, neurotmesis or axonotmesis to the brachial plexus; second, avulsion of the nerve roots from the spinal cord.

3. (a) **True**
   (b) **True**
   (c) **False**
   (d) **True**
   (e) **True**

Electrophysiological studies may be of considerable help in localizing the site of the lesion. The axon reflex is lost when the lesion is distal to the dorsal root ganglion but is preserved when the lesion lies proximally and would therefore be expected to be present in this case, certainly within C8 and T1. The distal connections with the dorsal root ganglion are also required for the detection of the sensory nerve action potential and in lesions involving the brachial plexus or a peripheral nerve this would be expected to be lost. Motor conduction velocities would be expected to be normal and at 3 weeks it is too early for the changes of denervation to be seen in muscles which may be electrically silent. 'F' waves tend to reflect proximal conduction within the arm, provided that the peripheral nerve was intact, and would be expected to be preserved in intact segments.

Questions

4. What investigation does *Figure 9a* depict, and what does it suggest?

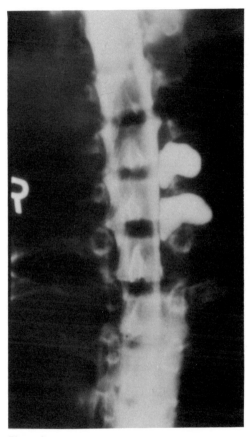

Figure 9a

5. What is the prognosis for recovery?

Answers

4. *Figure 9a* is a myelogram showing meningoceles at C7, C8 and T1, suggesting that avulsion of the nerve roots has occurred at these levels.
5. Provided that there is evidence of innervation there is potential for recovery. When the lesion can be localized to the brachial plexus it is possible to re-establish continuity by nerve grafting, although regeneration takes place only slowly. When avulsion has occurred no recovery is possible and consideration must therefore be given to amputation and construction of a limb prosthesis.

Comment

Investigation showed that he had traumatic avulsion of C7, C8 and T1. Little recovery was made, although there was a preserved axon reflex in C5 and 6 and he made some recovery in muscles innervated by these nerve roots.

Further reading

SEDDON, H., *Surgical Disorders of the Peripheral Nerves* (1975), Churchill Livingstone, Edinburgh, 179 *et seq.*

Case 9.5 Acute paraparesis

A 48-year-old woman was admitted with a 4-day history of increasing weakness in both lower limbs, together with a feeling of tightness and band-like constriction of both ankles. At the time of onset of the symptoms she had acute mid-dorsal pain without radiation lasting for approximately 30 min. In the 24 h before admission, there had been disturbance of bladder function and she had been incontinent of urine. There was no significant previous history and, in particular, no history of diplopia, visual disturbance, dizziness or speech disturbance and no previous history of abnormalities in function of any limb. She had suffered a mild, uncomplicated, upper respiratory tract infection 10 days before admission.

On examination there was no visible abnormality over the dorsal spine and no spinal tenderness. Cranial nerves and upper limbs were normal. She had a flaccid paraparesis with retained knee and ankle jerks; plantar reflexes were extensor; abdominal reflexes were absent. There was a sensory level to all modalities bilaterally at D6 with involvement of the sacral dermatomes. The bladder was palpable at the umbilicus.

Questions

1. Which of the following diagnoses should be considered:

    (a) Tumour metastasis in the lumbar region?
    (b) Postinfective polyneuropathy (Guillain–Barré syndrome)?
    (c) Multiple sclerosis?
    (d) Anterior spinal artery occlusion?
    (e) Postviral transverse myelitis?

2. What investigations should be undertaken?

3. What treatment is indicated?

4. What is the prognosis?

Answers

1. (a) **False**
   (b) **False**
   (c) **True**
   (d) **False**
   (e) **True**

The clinical signs suggest an acute lesion at D6. Anterior spinal artery occlusion would be associated with a dissociated sensory loss, i.e. retained dorsal column modalities. A postinfective polyneuropathy can present acutely but severe sensory symptoms and retention of urine would be unusual and the tendon reflexes would be lost. Transverse myelitis can follow a viral infection or be the presenting feature of multiple sclerosis.

2. Dorsal spine radiography, myelography and CSF examination including immunoglobulin studies.

3. Steroids are usually given to reduce spinal cord oedema associated with acute demyelination and may improve the ultimate outcome.

4. In transverse myelitis about 30% recover completely, 30% are partially disabled, and 30% do not recover. It is important to protect skin, avoid bladder infection and constipation, and prevent muscle spasms and consequent contractures.

Comment

Dorsal spine radiography and the myelogram were normal. CSF was under opening pressure of 180 mm and was clear; protein was 1.2 g/l with 20% IgG and no oligoclonal banding; glucose was 3.5 mmol/l (blood glucose 5.0 mmol/l). There were 50 reactive lymphocytes/µl. The patient was thought to have an acute postviral transverse myelitis. Recovery was slow but 1 year after the onset she was walking with a stick and had regained urinary continence.

Further reading

MATTHEWS, W. B. (ed), *McAlpine's Multiple Sclerosis* (1985), Churchill Livingstone, Edinburgh

Case 9.6 Coma of uncertain origin

A 42-year-old man was found unconscious at home. No other history was available. He was emaciated with 12 spider naevi over the trunk. External examination of the skull was normal and there was no neck stiffness. He was breathing regularly at a rate of 20/min and his breath had a distinctive musty smell. Pulse rate was 75/min and blood pressure was 120/80 mmHg. To a painful stimulus the patient did not open his eyes but he groaned; to supraorbital pressure he grimaced and both arms extended. The pupils were 4 mm in diameter and reacted briskly to light. When the eyelids were held open, the eyes were divergent and roving randomly in a dysconjugate fashion. Rotation of the head to each side was associated with deviation of the eyes to the opposite side (preserved doll's head manoeuvre or oculocephalic reflex). Corneal reflexes were brisk. There was a mild increase in tone in the limbs. Tendon stretch reflexes were brisk. There was sustained ankle clonus bilaterally and the plantar reflexes were extensor.

Questions

1. The following concerning the clinical signs may be true or false:

   (a) Preserved pupillary reflexes exclude a brain-stem lesion.
   (b) Extensor motor responses indicate brain-stem disease.
   (c) Dysconjugate eyes indicate bilateral VIth nerve palsies.
   (d) Ankle clonus indicates a spinal cord lesion.
   (e) Bilateral grimace responses suggest psychogenic coma.

Answers

1. (a) **False**
   (b) **False**
   (c) **False**
   (d) **False**
   (e) **False**

Pupillary reflexes are mediated through the IIIrd cranial nerve at the level of the superior colliculus. A lower brain-stem lesion producing coma by damage to the reticular formation may not involve the pupillary reflexes, but if all the brain-stem reflexes are preserved this excludes a brain-stem lesion. Extensor motor responses (decerebrate posturing) have no anatomical correlate and may be seen in lesions in the brain stem, diencephalon or the cerebral hemispheres. Dysconjugate eyes in a patient in coma are of no particular significance. In normal sleep the eyes tend to be divergent and in light coma this is a common finding. In this case bilateral VIth nerve palsies are excluded by the full reflex eye movement. Ankle clonus and extensor plantar reflexes confirm pyramidal tract involvement but do not indicate the level. A grimace response is a motor response of the facial muscles to a painful stimulus; it occurs in most comatose patients who move their arms in response to pain and is of no particular diagnostic significance. In psychogenic coma the caloric reflexes produce normal nystagmus. In this patient tonic caloric reflexes exclude psychogenic coma.

Questions

2. Which of the following diagnoses should be considered:
   (a) Subdural haematoma?
   (b) Subarachnoid haemorrhage?
   (c) Drug overdose?
   (d) Encephalitis?
   (e) Hepatic encephalopathy?

Answers

2. (a) **False**
   (b) **False**
   (c) **False**
   (d) **True**
   (e) **True**

Pathophysiologically, three types of coma are recognized: (i) brain-stem coma; (ii) coma due to unilateral hemisphere lesion with 'coning', in which coma occurs as rostrocaudal herniation and distortion of the brain stem disrupts the reticular formation, resulting in asymmetrical brain-stem reflexes, cranial nerve palsies and limb responses; (iii) cerebral hemisphere coma. Absence of focal signs and symmetrical brisk brain-stem reflexes make (i) and (ii) unlikely, and suggest that coma is due to bilateral depression of cerebral hemisphere function. Common causes are subarachnoid haemorrhage, diffuse cerebral anoxia, metabolic insults and meningitis or encephalitis. Subdural haematoma is unlikely as most patients unconscious due to subdural haematoma have focal signs. Absence of meningeal irritation makes subarachnoid haemorrhage most unlikely. Although neck stiffness may be absent in unresponsive flaccid patients, those in light coma, i.e. those who respond to pain, would be expected to have neck stiffness as they retain muscle tone. Drug coma is associated with selective depression of brain-stem reflexes, particularly reflex eye movement; brisk brain-stem reflexes in this patient exclude drug coma. Although possible, encephalitis is unlikely in the absence of fits, focal signs, fever or neck stiffness. One of the commonest forms of metabolic coma is that seen in patients with hepatic failure and the signs in this case would be entirely compatible with this diagnosis. The foetor and spider naevi are further clues to the diagnosis.

Question

3. What are the priorities of management?

Answers

3. The following are important priorities in management:

   (a) Maintain airway and vital functions including ventilation and circulation.
   (b) Obtain information about a diagnosis, including history from relatives, ambulance drivers, police and any documents that the patient may be carrying.
   (c) Serial assessment of conscious level to assess whether the patient is getting better or worse.
   (d) Investigations including blood glucose to exclude hypoglycaemia, and cranial CT if there are localizing signs to suggest a mass lesion or hydrocephalus.

Comment

In this case CT was normal. Information became available concerning the patient's previous history and it was discovered that he had previously been investigated for alcoholic liver disease in another hospital. Haematological and biochemical investigations were compatible with the diagnosis of hepatic coma and, with appropriate treatment, he recovered.

Further reading

PLUM, F. and POSNER, J. B., 'Multifocal, diffuse and metabolic brain diseases causing stupor and coma', *The Diagnosis of Stupor and Coma*, 3rd edition (1985), F. A. Davis Co., Philadelphia, Chapter 4

Exercise 10

Case 10.1 A stroke in a 17-year-old girl

A 17-year-old girl visited her general practitioner in a very distressed state because she suddenly experienced difficulty in speaking and thought that she had had a stroke. The previous night, pain in and around the left ear had been sufficient to keep her awake and that morning her mouth had become twisted. Looking in the mirror she noticed that her left eye did not close and, when she was washing, the eye became red and sore and watered continuously. Taste and hearing were normal.

Neurological examination revealed a complete paralysis of the left-sided facial muscles.

Questions

1. (a) What is the most probable diagnosis?
   (b) What other functions should be examined?
   (c) What investigations are indicated?
   (d) What treatment is indicated?

Answers

1. (a) Bell's palsy.
   (b) Tearing: the parasympathetic supply to the lacrimal gland passes with the VIIth cranial nerve in its subarachnoid portion before joining the greater superficial petrosal nerve. Damage proximal to the geniculate ganglion is associated with loss of tearing.
   Taste: the chorda tympani conveys taste from the anterior two-thirds of the tongue.
   Hearing: the nerve to stapedius exits from the VIIth cranial nerve proximal to the foramen spinosum. Loss of taste and hyperacusis imply a lesion proximal to the foramen spinosum in the intracanalicular portion of the nerve.
   (c) No investigations are indicated unless there is evidence that the lesion lies in the subarachnoid space, i.e. tearing is lost. Subacute meningitis due to leukaemia, lymphoma, sarcoid, cancer or chronic infection should then be excluded.
   (d) Corticosteroids, if used early, may improve the prognosis.

Steroids were given for one month without improvement. After 3 months she thought that the eye was closing and sought further advice.

On examination, the eye on the affected side appeared to be closing and the eyelid moved when she was eating, talking or smiling. There was a facial contracture on the affected side. The palpebral fissure was narrow and there was a mild degree of weakness; the patient could close her eye and smile. When asked to blink there was a contraction of mentalis; when asked to purse her lips there was contraction of the periorbital facial muscles resulting in eye closure. Forced eye opening revealed the globe to be elevated.

Questions

2. (a) What has occurred?
   (b) What is the prognosis for further recovery?
   (c) What treatment can be given?

Answers

2. (a) She has a facial contracture which, in patients in whom little motor recovery takes place, may improve the cosmetic appearance of the face. She also has a synkinesis due to aberrant regeneration of the facial nerve, so that fibres destined for the upper facial muscle have reinnervated those of the lower face and vice versa. Elevation of the globe on forced eye closure is physiological (Bell's phenomenon).

   (b) The prognosis for further recovery is poor because regrowth has already occurred.

   (c) No treatment is available other than reassurance.

Comment

A 17-year-old girl presented with Bell's palsy. Recovery was delayed despite steroids and resulted in aberrant regeneration and a facial synkinesis.

Further reading

DYCK, P. J., THOMAS, P. K. and LAMBERT, E. H., 'Bell's palsy', *Peripheral Neuropathy* (1975), W. B. Saunders, Philadelphia, 585

Case 10.2   A lump on the head

A 75-year-old woman was noted by her hairdresser to have a lump on her head. Her general practitioner described a large round smooth and firm lump over the vertex, and sent her to a neurologist. Ten years previously the patient had a single grand mal convulsion, and subsequently she had had infrequent partial seizures, not controlled by a small dose of phenobarbitone. Over the previous year she had been noted by her relatives to have become increasingly forgetful and also at times a little unsteady with a tendency to stumble.

Examination confirmed the presence of a mass on the skull as described by the GP. There was mild impairment of cognition. She had a pout reflex, generally brisk tendon stretch reflexes, and a mild gait ataxia.

Questions

1. What is the probable diagnosis?
2. What is the relevance of the history of epilepsy?
3. Why is she ataxic and mildly demented?

Answers

1. She has a 'mushroom meningioma', a parasagittal tumour eroding through the skull with both an intracranial and an extracranial component.
2. She has partial and secondarily generalized epilepsy as a result of the tumour.
3. A large supratentorial tumour or hydrocephalus may cause 'frontal lobe' ataxia and dementia.

It was not thought possible to remove the tumour surgically and she was treated with phenytoin sodium. She lived a relatively normal life for the next 2 years but was admitted to hospital having gone into status epilepticus from which she never recovered, dying within 12 h of admission.

Comment

Erosion through the skull produces an effective decompression of the intracranial compartment and will reduce the likelihood of signs due to cerebral compression. Involvement of the skull by meningiomas is by no means rare, and makes the tumour difficult to remove completely, increasing the chance of a recurrence.

Further reading

RICHENS, A., 'Treatment of status epilepticus', *Drug Treatment of Epilepsy* (1976), Henry Kimpton, London, 96

Case 10.3 Pes cavus

A 19-year-old right-handed secretary was referred by the Orthopaedic Department for assessment before an operation for bilateral pes cavus. She had always known about an abnormality affecting her feet and claimed that she had never been good at games at school. She used to avoid physical education whenever possible and was not as agile as her peers. In the previous 12 months she had twisted her ankle and fallen because her walking had deteriorated. She was unsteady and clumsy, especially in the dark, and her feet had become numb. Her hands were normal and she had passed her typing examinations with moderate grades and was capable in her present job as a secretary. There was no sphincter disturbance. Her father was wheelchair bound with an illness diagnosed as a form of muscular dystrophy. Her paternal aunt and the aunt's son had similar foot deformities and had walking difficulties which began in their early 20s. The patient's brother had high arched feet and was poor at physical activities.

The legs were wasted with an 'inverted champagne bottle' appearance. There was bilateral pes cavus. The spine appeared normal. No peripheral nerves were palpable. Tone was flaccid and the tendon stretch reflexes absent. Distal muscles in the legs were weak, especially in dorsiflexion and eversion at the ankle. There was a lesser degree of weakness in the arms. There was sensory loss in all modalities to the knees bilaterally. Cranial nerves were normal.

Questions

1. The following concerning the disorder may be true or false:

   (a) Spina bifida may be the cause of this patient's symptoms.
   (b) The pattern of inheritance is that of muscular dystrophy.
   (c) The findings are those of a chronic peripheral neuropathy.
   (d) Vitamin B_{12} deficiency is a probable cause of this syndrome.
   (e) The patient may have porphyria.

Answers

1. (a) **False**
   (b) **False**
   (c) **True**
   (d) **False**
   (e) **False**

Mixed motor and sensory symptoms, gradually progressing first in the legs and then the arms, with a family history which suggests a dominant pattern of inheritance would be compatible with chronic sensorimotor neuropathy of the Charcot–Marie–Tooth variety (peroneal muscular atrophy or Type 1 Hereditary Sensorimotor Neuropathy). Patients with spina bifida usually have bladder and bowel involvement. Subacute combined degeneration of the cord presents commonly with a shorter history and sensory symptoms beginning in the upper limbs. The neuropathy of porphyria is mainly motor and not associated with skeletal abnormalities. Most cases of muscular dystrophy have a recessive pattern of inheritance.

Question

2. The following concerning investigations may be true or false:

    (a) Muscle biopsy is indicated.
    (b) Nerve conduction velocity would be expected to be slowed.
    (c) Nerve biopsy is indicated to exclude Refsum's disease.

Answers

2. (a) **False**
   (b) **True**
   (c) **False**

Investigations should identify the type of neuropathy and its cause. Nerve conduction studies and electromyography may distinguish between an axonal and demyelinating neuropathy, conduction velocity being slowed in the latter. Muscle biopsy would show changes of denervation in patients with neurogenic disorder but is usually only indicated in patients with primary muscle disease. Nerve biopsy would be expected to show demyelination with remyelination – the 'onion bulb' appearance responsible for producing nerve hypertrophy – although this need not be present clinically. Refsum's disease can be adequately excluded by assay of serum phytanic acid; in this patient, the dominant pattern of inheritance, and lack of deafness, retinitis pigmentosa or a skin rash, make this diagnosis untenable.

Comment

Routine haematological and biochemical tests were normal. Nerve conduction velocity was 25 m/s. This patient's investigations, including nerve biopsy, indicated that she had a chronic neuropathy of the Charcot–Marie–Tooth variety (Type 1, Hereditary Sensorimotor Neuropathy. Pes cavus not infrequently is secondary to neurological diseases such as a chronic sensorimotor neuropathy.

Further reading

DYCK, P. J., THOMAS, P. K. and LAMBERT, H. E. H., *Peripheral Neuropathy* (1975), W. B. Saunders, Philadelphia, Chapter 41

Case 10.4 Painful ophthalmoplegia

A 64-year-old woman presented to the Out-Patient Department with a history of pain in the left eye, double vision and drooping of the left eyelid. Six months previously she developed pain in and around the left eye, which she described as throbbing in character. The pain increased in severity to the extent that it kept her awake at night and she needed to take larger doses of analgesics. After 3 months she noticed double vision on gaze to the left, which gradually became more marked. In the previous 4 weeks the left eyelid had drooped and this gradually increased in severity so that eventually the eye closed. On examination she appeared healthy, although she was obviously in pain. Blood pressure was 160/80 mmHg. There was complete left ptosis and, when the eyelid was elevated, the left pupil was seen to be dilated. When a light was shone in either eye, only the right pupil constricted and the left remained dilated. Movements of the right eye were normal, but the patient could not move the left eye in any direction. The left corneal reflex was absent.

Questions

1. The following concerning the physical signs may be true or false:

   (a) A bruit heard over the left orbit would suggest an underlying caroticocavernous fistula.
   (b) The pupillary changes suggest involvement of the left optic nerve.
   (c) An absent corneal reflex indicates trigeminal nerve involvement.
   (d) Ptosis suggests involvement of the VIIth cranial nerve.
   (e) The eye movement disorder suggests that the IVth nerve is intact.

2. Which of the following are probable anatomical sites for the lesion:

   (a) The orbit?
   (b) The anterior cranial fossa?
   (c) Near the cavernous sinus?
   (d) Within the brain stem?
   (e) In the region of the clivus?

Answers

1. (a) **False**
   (b) **False**
   (c) **True**
   (d) **False**
   (e) **False**

The signs are those of a complete ophthalmoplegia due to involvement of the IIIrd, IVth and VIth cranial nerves. IVth nerve function (superior oblique) is normally tested by asking the patient to look down with the eye adducted; in the presence of a IIIrd nerve palsy, however, the IVth nerve causes the eye to intort and may be tested by asking the patient to look down with the eye in abduction. Pupillary changes are those of a IIIrd nerve palsy: the pupil does not react either directly or consensually. If the IInd nerve were involved, then neither pupil would react to light in the ipsilateral eye, but both would react to light in the contralateral eye. An absent corneal reflex indicates involvement of the ophthalmic division of the Vth nerve. Ptosis results from weakness of levator palpebrae superioris, innervated by the IIIrd cranial nerve and the cervical sympathetic nerves and in this case is due to a IIIrd nerve lesion. Patients with a VIIth nerve lesion, e.g. Bell's palsy, do not have ptosis. A bruit may be heard over a caroticocavernous fistula but it is invariably associated with proptosis and hyperaemia of the conjunctiva, both of which are absent. In this patient a bruit would indicate turbulent blood flow in or around the orbit and would be compatible with either a vascular tumour or a lesion involving the carotid siphon.

2. (a) **False**
   (b) **False**
   (c) **True**
   (d) **False**
   (e) **True**

The probable site of pathological changes in this case is the parasellar region near or in the cavernous sinus. The IIIrd, IVth and VIth cranial nerves and the first division of the Vth cranial nerves all pass together over the clivus and through the cavernous sinus to the orbit. Lesions in the orbit and anterior cranial fossa also involve the IInd cranial nerve and cause proptosis. Brain-stem lesions involve either the ascending or descending motor and sensory pathways.

Questions

3. Which of the following are probable pathological causes:

    (a) A glioma?
    (b) An aneurysm?
    (c) A meningioma?
    (d) A metastasis?
    (e) A mucocele?

Answers

3. (a) **False**
   (b) **True**
   (c) **True**
   (d) **True**
   (e) **True**

The lesion is lying outside the substance of the brain. An aneurysm or a meningioma in the cavernous sinus may cause this syndrome. Intracavernous aneurysms typically compress the IIIrd, IVth and VIth cranial nerves and also may involve the first and rarely the second divisions of the Vth nerve. They tend to occur in older patients and are characterized by pain, tending to progress over weeks or months. Meningiomas in the region of the cavernous sinus more commonly involve the IInd cranial nerve, producing visual loss, and are typically painless. less likely is a metastasis or mucocele. A metastasis or nasopharyngeal tumour is usually painful, and an ethmoid sinus mucocele usually causes proptosis.

Questions

4. Which of the following are possible methods of treatment in this case:

   (a) Left common carotid ligation?
   (b) Radiotherapy?
   (c) Direct clipping of the aneurysm?
   (d) Treatment with ε-aminocaproic acid?

Answers

4. (a) **True**
   (b) **False**
   (c) **False**
   (d) **False**

Treatment of intracavernous aneurysm is difficult and a variety of methods have been used. The main indication for treatment is pain, as cranial nerve palsies rarely recover. Clipping is technically difficult because aneurysms are merely fusiform dilatations of the carotid artery. Carotid ligation will relieve pain but there is a risk of stroke which may be partially overcome by superficial temporal–middle cerebral artery anastomosis before surgery. Neither conventional radiotherapy nor antifibrinolytic therapy, e.g. ε-aminocaproic acid, has any place in the management of these aneurysms.

Comment

Intracavernous aneurysms rarely rupture; if they do, they are most likely to rupture into the cavernous sinus, producing a caroticocavernous fistula. In this patient an intracavernous aneurysm presenting with painful ophthalmoplegia was treated by ligation of the common carotid artery, with good pain relief. Chest and skull radiographs were normal. Cranial CT showed a high-attenuation lesion in the left parasellar region; carotid angiography confirmed this to be an intracavernous aneurysm.

Further reading

BARR, H. W. K., BLACKWOOD, W. and MEADOWS, S. P., 'Intracavernous carotid aneurysms. A clinico pathological report', *Brain* (1977), **94**, 607

Case 10.5 Progressively impaired consciousness

A 45-year-old woman collapsed in the street. She had previously been healthy, apart from shortness of breath when walking up stairs or up inclines. As a young girl she had had an illness that was diagnosed as rheumatic fever but she had not been examined since and had not sought any medical attention.

On admission she was alert and opened her eyes to command. She was able to utter occasional sounds but produced no recognizable words. She was unable to understand other than the most simple commands such as 'close your eyes; open your mouth'. She had a complete right homonymous hemianopia and a flaccid paralysis of the right arm. There was some minimal movement of the right leg. Tendon stretch reflexes in the right arm were absent and in the leg appeared equal to those on the left. There was no plantar reflex on the right. Sensory testing was difficult because of her inability to comprehend commands. However, she appeared to have dense sensory loss on the right side of her body to the extent that even an extremely painful stimulus did not produce any obvious response. The pulse was irregular. The heart was enlarged and there was a loud mid-diastolic murmur audible at the apex.

Questions

1. What is the anatomical basis of the abnormal neurological signs?
2. What is the pathological basis?
3. What is the management?

Over the next few hours the patient's level of consciousness began to deteriorate and when she became drowsy, her eyes drifted conjugately to the left. Her eyes opened to a painful stimulus and the right arm extended, but the right leg showed little response to pain.

4. What is the mechanism of her deterioration?
5. Can anything be done to prevent further deterioration?

Answers

1. The signs indicate a large lesion involving the left hemisphere including the internal capsule and possibly the thalamus.
2. The sudden onset of an extensive cerebral hemisphere lesion with preserved consciousness suggests infarction; the presence of the atrial fibrillation and signs suggesting mitral stenosis would suggest that this has resulted from an embolus, probably in the middle cerebral artery.
3. Management of an infarct is controversial. There is no specific treatment that is likely to help the area of infarction, although anticoagulants may prevent further episodes. There is a risk, however, that they would cause haemorrhage into the infarct.
4. Signs now suggest that rostrocaudal herniation is occurring due to cerebral oedema. Conjugate deviation of the eyes is a common finding in an acute hemisphere stroke, and is evidence of a supranuclear gaze palsy resulting from hemisphere damage.
5. Cranial CT should be performed to exclude primary intra-cerebral haemorrhage; in this patient it showed a large low-attenuation lesion in the left hemisphere, assumed to be infarction with surrounding oedema.

Comment

There is no effective treatment for ischaemic cerebral oedema. It is likely that herniation will continue and that the patient will die as a result. Mannitol, dexamethasone and a variety of other medications have been used, but none are of proven value. The prognosis for massive hemisphere infarction is appalling, most deaths resulting from brain swelling due to cerebral oedema, for which no treatment is available.

Further reading

PLUM, F. and POSNER, J. B., 'Supratentorial lesions causing coma', *The Diagnosis of Stupor and Coma* (1980), F. A. Davis Co., Philadelphia, Chapter 3

Case 10.6 Acute confusion after an operation

A medical registrar was summoned to examine a man on a surgical ward because of acute confusion. The patient was a 52-year-old garage proprietor who had had indigestion for many years and had been admitted to the surgical ward 3 days previously with a perforated duodenal ulcer.

Apart from the signs of an acute abdomen, examination was unremarkable except for the absence of the ankle jerks. Preliminary screening investigations were normal and an emergency laparotomy was performed. A perforated duodenal ulcer was treated by oversewing. Initial postoperative recovery was satisfactory but on the second day the patient was found to be slightly confused and during the following night he became irrational, was shouting and tried to get out of bed. Nursing staff had difficulty in controlling him and a Medical Consultation was sought.

The medical registrar who examined the patient found him to be tremulous. Temperature was 38.4°C. Pulse was 125/min, blood pressure 120/90 mmHg. He was irrational and uncooperative and was difficult to examine. He frequently plucked at his bedclothes and pointed around the room as if able to see objects that were not present. No focal neurological abnormality was detected, although the registrar confirmed the absence of ankle reflexes.

Questions

1. (a) What is the probable diagnosis?
   (b) What further questions should be asked?
   (c) What investigations should be performed?
   (d) What treatment should be given?
   (e) What is the prognosis?

Answers

1. (a) Acute confusion with tremulousness and visual halluci-
       nations beginning 3 days after admission to hospital
       suggests delirium tremens.
   (b) The patient's wife should be questioned about her husband's
       alcohol intake. This revealed that he had consumed large
       quantities of beer and spirits for many years.
   (c) No specific investigations are required other than those to
       demonstrate further damage due to alcohol excess, e.g.
       MCV and liver function tests.
   (d) Treatment is by sedation using either a benzodiazepine or
       chlormethiazole.
   (e) Delirium tremens is a self-limiting condition; although
       occasionally patients may die from exhaustion, with sedation
       most patients recover.

The patient was given a chlormethiazole infusion and sedated to the extent that he was no longer noisy and restless. Tremulousness improved and over the next 24 h temperature and tachycardia, a feature of delirium tremens, settled. Confusion, however, persisted and the patient developed nystagmus in all directions of gaze and his speech became slurred. The medical registrar thought this was due to chlormethiazole but requested that his consultant examine the patient. The physician confirmed the signs, including confusion, nystagmus and dysarthria, but noted in addition that the patient had some impairment of upward conjugate gaze. He suggested an alternative diagnosis.

Questions

2. (a) What is the alternative diagnosis?
   (b) What treatment should be given?
   (c) What is the prognosis?

Answers

2. (a) Wernicke–Korsakoff syndrome.
   (b) This is due to thiamine deficiency; the patient should be given 200 mg thiamine daily, without which he may die,
   (c) With treatment the prognosis is quite good, although confusion may take some weeks to clear. As many as one-third of patients will be left with permanent memory defects, including confabulation. Treatment with thiamine should continue indefinitely.

Comment

Neurological complications of alcoholism are often missed as patients frequently do not admit to their habits. In this patient the only clue was absent ankle jerks due to a subclinical peripheral neuropathy. Delirium tremens typically develops in someone with a high alcohol intake for many years, who is then suddenly withdrawn from alcohol, and it should enter the differential diagnosis of a sudden episode of confusion in a recently hospitalized patient. Anyone with a known high alcohol intake should routinely be given sedatives on admission to hospital to prevent delirium tremens. If it occurs, patients should be treated with multivitamin preparations containing thiamine to prevent the Wernicke–Korsakoff syndrome. This commonly presents following an episode of delirium tremens and may be precipitated by a surgical procedure. Confusion is a prominent feature but the diagnosis is strengthened by the finding of signs of a brain-stem disturbance such as nystagmus, supranuclear eye-movement disorders, ataxia and dysarthria.

Further reading

VICTOR, M., ADAMS, R. D. and COLLINS, G. H. (eds), *The Wernicke–Korsakoff Syndrome* (1973), F. A. Davis Co., Philadelphia

Exercise 11

Case 11.1 Deterioration after head injury

A 26-year-old woman was hit by a car when crossing a road. When the ambulance arrived she was awake and talking, but appeared confused and complained of headache. On arrival at the Accident and Emergency Department she was alert and able to answer questions, but still occasionally appeared confused and continued to complain of quite severe headache. No abnormal neurological signs were detected. Skull radiography showed a left parietal fracture. The patient reached the ward 2½ h after the accident and gave the house officer a clear history of events following arrival at hospital. She still complained of a severe headache and was rubbing the left side of her head. Shortly after admission to the ward she vomited. Half an hour later when her relatives arrived at the hospital she was drowsy and slow in talking to them; 15 min later, she had to be aroused by shaking and was very slow to answer questions. The house officer confirmed this. Only an extensor right-sided plantar reflex was found.

Questions

1. The following concerning this patient may be true or false:

    (a) Left-sided headache is likely to be due to scalp lacerations.
    (b) Extensor plantars suggest a cervical cord injury.
    (c) Drowsiness suggests concussion.
    (d) The skull fracture may safely be ignored.
    (e) She should be sedated and left to sleep.

2. Which of the following should be undertaken:

    (a) Treatment with high-dose steroids?
    (b) Cranial CT?
    (c) Carotid angiography?
    (d) Left-sided burr holes?

Answers

1. (a) **False**
   (b) **False**
   (c) **False**
   (d) **False**
   (e) **False**

Without urgent treatment this patient was likely to die. Signs suggested a left-sided extradural haematoma with rostrocaudal herniation. Headache and left-sided scalp irritation suggested the site of the haematoma. Drowsiness suggested increased ICP and the extensor plantar response on the right was due to uncal herniation.

2. (a) **False**
   (b) **True**
   (c) **False**
   (d) **True**

Cranial CT, carotid angiography or a diagnostic burr hole may be done to confirm the diagnosis. A burr hole is associated with a higher mortality than CT: if there is cerebral oedema, the brain may herniate. Steroids would not be indicated.

Cranial CT confirmed the presence of a left-sided extradural haematoma which was drained and bleeding meningeal vessels ligated. After surgery the patient regained consciousness and by the next day she was up and about the ward, talking normally.

Comment

Extradural haematomas in young people are characteristically associated with an ipsilateral skull fracture and develop within 6–24 h of the trauma. Extradural haematoma is a complication of the skull, not brain, injury.

Further reading

JENNETT, B. AND TEASDALE, G., 'Intracranial haematoma', (1980), *Management of Head Injuries*. F. A. Davies Co., Philadelphia, Chapter 7

Case 11.2 Sudden visual loss

A 65-year-old man presented to the Out-Patient Department with recurrent attacks of loss of vision in the left eye. The first was 6 months previously when a black area gradually descended like a curtain to occlude vision completely in the left eye. Vision was impaired for a few minutes and then the curtain gradually rose and vision returned to normal. Since then, 10–15 similar attacks had occurred, none of which appeared to have been precipitated by any specific activity. Apart from chest pain brought on by exertion, the patient was healthy.

Examination revealed a plethoric man. Blood pressure was 130/70 mmHg, cardiac examination was normal. Auscultation of the neck revealed a loud bruit over the left angle of the jaw. Neurological examination was normal.

Questions

1. What is this visual phenomenon?
2. What is the differential diagnosis?
3. What is the significance of the bruit?
4. What is the prognosis?

Answers

1. Amaurosis fugax.
2. Although retinal emboli are the probable cause, low flow states induced by carotid occlusion, ophthalmic artery aneurysm and glaucoma should be considered.
3. It is suggestive of symptomatic carotid artery stenosis.
4. Approximately 5% of patients with amaurosis fugax have a hemisphere or retinal stroke, although it is likely that the risk is maximal in the first year.

Comment

Amaurosis fugax is often attributable to retinal emboli arising from carotid stenosis. Current evidence suggests that patients are at risk from stroke and should be treated as for cerebral transient ischaemic attacks (Case 12.6). The neuropathies associated with diabetes, amyloid and porphyria and the Guillan Barre Syndrome most characteristically affect autonomic function.

Further reading

MARSHALL, J. and MEADOWS, S., 'The natural history of amaurosis fugax', *Brain* (1968), **91**, 419

Case 11.3 Dizzy spells

A 56-year-old vicar was sent to hospital by his general practitioner for investigation of fainting spells. For 5 years he had had an increasing tendency to faint on standing. He often experienced premonitory symptoms of dizziness and haziness of vision and occasionally he could prevent himself from fainting by sitting down. Initially, the dizziness was most marked in the mornings but, as time went by, any standing produced the premonitory symptoms and if he remained erect for more than a few minutes he was likely to faint. Because of this he had had to curtail his activities severely and he was only able to walk a few steps before he had to sit down.

When, aged 30 years, he was on holiday in Greece for the first time, he became ill during the second week and was treated in hospital for what he was told was heat stroke. Over the next few years he became aware that he could not tolerate being in hot environments for prolonged periods and he had to stop taking holidays abroad in hot climates. At the age of 40 years he became impotent and by his late 40s he began to develop symptoms of frequency of micturition which, within a year or two was accompanied by urge incontinence. At that time he also became aware of a tendency to chronic constipation.

In his early 50s he began to notice unsteadiness of gait, separate from the dizziness. Initially, after the equivalent of only one or two drinks, he would become unsteady and would slur his speech. With time this unsteadiness and slurred speech had increased and was noticeable even without alcohol ingestion. Because of all these symptoms he had had to conduct services sitting down.

Examination revealed a healthy man who immediately on standing became pale and complained of feeling unwell. Pulse was 62/min and regular and did not appear to vary when lying, sitting or standing. Lying blood pressure was 129/80 mmHg, sitting was 95/70 mmHg and standing was 60/20 mmHg and then unrecordable. His skin was dry. He was dysarthric and had a truncal ataxia. Dizziness prevented him from walking. There was a minor degree of incoordination in the limbs; tendon stretch reflexes were brisk.

Questions

1. What is the significance of the following groups of symptoms:

    (a) Heat intolerance?
    (b) Dizziness induced on standing?
    (c) Urge incontinence and constipation?
    (d) Impotence?

2. What is the significance of these signs:

    (a) Fixed pulse rate?
    (b) Orthostatic hypotension?
    (c) Signs of cerebellar ataxia?

Answers

1. Each of these symptoms is compatible with autonomic failure.

2. (a, b) The fixed pulse rate and orthostatic hypotension suggest autonomic failure. There is evidence of sympathetic and parasympathetic failure. Orthostatic hypotension indicates sympathetic failure and loss of the sinus arrhythmia, incontinence and constipation suggest parasympathetic failure. Heat stroke and heat intolerance are unusual symptoms but are occasionally seen in patients who have lost thermoregulation.

   (c) They suggest that the cerebellar connections are also involved and that this is a systems degeneration with autonomic and cerebellar involvement.

Questions

3. What is the diagnosis?
4. What investigations are indicated?
5. What forms of treatment may be offered?

Answers

3. Multisystem atrophy or the Shy–Drager syndrome.

4. Investigations should be directed towards confirming the diagnosis and the degree of autonomic involvement. Absence of thermoregulatory sweating can be tested by raising the patient's body temperature by 1°C. Parasympathetic function may be assessed using the sinus arrhythmia, the heart rate response to a Valsalva manoeuvre, and standing. The blood pressure response to standing and sustained hand grip is a measure of sympathetic function.

5. The prognosis is appalling. The condition is likely to progress and result in the patient being incapacitated, chair-bound and eventually bed-bound. Ultimately patients succumb to pneumonia or a cardiac dysrhythmia. Various drugs have been used to treat orthostatic hypotension including a high salt diet, salt-retaining steroids, sympathetic agents, monoamamine oxidase inhibitors (and Marmite), pindolol, indomethacin, caffeine and ergotamine. None are particularly helpful, although they may produce a transient improvement in symptoms.

Comment

The Shy–Drager syndrome is a progressive disorder associated with degeneration of the central and peripheral autonomic nervous system and various other central nervous structures, particularly the cerebellum and vagal nucleus. Occasionally patients with multiple sclerosis may show evidence of a degree of autonomic neuropathy but, although this may be associated with impotence and bladder and bowel problems, it rarely produces orthostatic hypotension. Progressive autonomic failure is a feature of a number of forms of peripheral neuropathy but these are usually clinically obvious. The neuropathies associated with diabetes, amyloid and porphyria most characteristically affect autonomic function.

Further reading

BANNISTER, R. and OPPENHEIMER, D. R., 'Degenerative diseases of the nervous system associated with autonomic failure', *Brain* (1972), **95**, 457

Case 11.4 Unsteadiness

A 57-year-old woman presented to the Out-Patient Department with a 1-year history of increasing unsteadiness. She was using two sticks to help her at home and had frequent falls. She admitted to slurring of speech and some clumsiness of the right arm.

On examination she walked with a wide stiff-legged gait. She was orientated in place and time and had a normal memory. She had sensorineural deafness on the right. The right corneal reflex was depressed compared with the left. The right arm was clumsy and tendon stretch reflexes brisk, but plantar reflexes were flexor.

Questions

1. What is the differential diagnosis of unsteadiness at this age?
2. What is the significance of the right-sided hearing loss and depressed corneal reflex?
3. What investigations are indicated?

Answers

1. (a) Posterior fossa tumour.
   (b) Cerebellar degeneration, although these usually progress slowly, other than certain forms of paraneoplastic cerebellar degeneration which may present with marked limb ataxia and dysarthria.
   (c) Extrapyramidal disorders.
   (d) Spinal cord disease before patients are aware of weak legs.
   (e) Frontal tumours producing an apraxia of gait, with or without hydrocephalus.

2. Hearing loss and a depressed corneal reflex are localizing signs and suggest a lesion in the cerebellopontine angle, involving the VIIIth and Vth cranial nerves respectively.

3. Radiographs of the skull with view of the internal auditory meati; cranial CT; audiometry and tests of vestibular function.

Cranial CT showed a large acoustic neuroma producing distortion of the brain stem.

Comment

Acoustic neuromas may present with hearing loss and Vth and VIIth cranial nerve signs. Some patients, however, present only when there is brain-stem distortion resulting in ataxia or raised intracranial pressure due to obstruction to the outflow of cerebrospinal fluid from the IVth ventricle.

Further reading

JENNETT, B. and GALBRAITH, S., 'Acoustic neuroma', *An Introduction to Neurosurgery* (1983), 4th edition, Heinemann, London, 148

Case 11.5 An acute confusional state

A 55-year-old man was sent to hospital as an emergency by his general practitioner with a provisional diagnosis of acute confusional state. Six months previously the patient was made redundant; subsequently he had increased his drinking, spending lunchtime and most of the evening in the local public house where he consumed about 4 pints of beer at lunchtime and 6–8 pints of beer in the evening. Forty-eight hours before admission, he woke in the morning and complained of feeling unwell. He remained unwell for most of the morning and just before lunch he vomited. In the afternoon, he was noticed by his wife to be confused and a little irrational. Through that night he was irritable and remained awake and restless. The next morning, he was noticed to be unsteady and his 'confusion' was more marked: he was sent to hospital.

At the time of admission he was apyrexial. Blood pressure was 180/100 mmHg. He was alert and awake but had no recognizable words and produced rambling speech. He was able to obey simple commands such as 'lift your arm in the air', but nothing more complex. His eyes were deviated to the left and he had no menace response on the right side. Examination of the optic fundi revealed a number of flame-shaped haemorrhages over both optic discs. When sitting he tended to fall to the right and he moved his right arm less than his left. The right plantar reflex was extensor.

Questions

1. What is the interpretation of the physical signs?
2. What is the differential diagnosis?

Answers

1. The combination of a right hemianopia with a right hemiparesis is strong evidence of a focal lesion in the left hemisphere. The rambling speech with poor comprehension suggests the patient is not confused but dysphasic and this is compatible with a left hemisphere lesion.

2. Factors which have to be taken into account when considering the differential diagnosis are:

   (a) History of previous alcohol intake.
   (b) Localizing signs of a left hemisphere lesion.
   (c) Fundal haemorrhages.

The localizing signs in an alert patient suggest a lesion intrinsic to the left hemisphere. Retinal haemorrhages suggest that it is haemorrhagic. The most likely diagnosis would be an intra-cerebral haemorrhage, or subarachnoid haemorrhage, although the absence of meningism would make the latter less likely. A subdural haematoma would have to be considered with the previous history of high alcohol intake, but dysphasia is uncommon in this condition and drowsiness is a prominent feature. Herpes simplex encephalitis may present acutely with impaired consciousness, seizures and focal signs.

Questions

3. What does the CT scan in *Figure 11a* show?

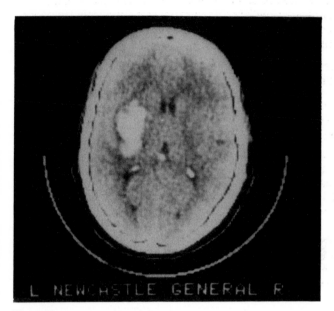

Figure 11a

4. What treatment should be given?
5. What is the prognosis for recovery?

Answers

3. A high attenuation lesion in the left temporal lobe suggesting an intracerebral haematoma.
4. Patients are best managed conservatively unless deteriorating rapidly. This patient should be sedated and treated with vitamins, including thiamine, in view of the previous history of a high alcohol intake.
5. Between 30% and 40% of patients with a haematoma die; however, functional recovery in survivors is better than in those with a cerebral infarct.

He was managed conservatively, sedated with chlormethiazole and given intravenous high-potency multivitamin preparations. His condition remained stable and then gradually improved over the next few weeks. He ultimately made a satisfactory recovery, being left with only mild word-finding difficulties.

Comment

This case illustrates that patients who survive an intracerebral haemorrhage may make quite a good functional recovery. Hypertensive intracerebral haemorrhages typically occur deep in the cerebral hemispheres and result from rupture of a Charcot-Bouchard aneurysm. More superficial haemorrhages, such as in this case, may occur from small arteriovenous malformations which may be demonstrated on angiography.

Further reading

KASE, C. S. and MOHR, J. P., 'General features of intracranial haemorrhage', (eds Barnett, H. J. M., Mohr, J. P., Stein, B. M. and Yatsu, F. M.), *Stroke. Pathophysiology, Diagnosis and Management* (1986), Churchill Livingstone, Edinburgh, Chapter 27

Case 11.6 Painful feet and hands

A 67-year-old man presented with an 18-month history of numbness and burning pain beginning in the soles and extending upwards. Similar symptoms had begun in the fingertips of both hands and spread to both wrists. Immediately before presentation he had been aware of an abnormal sensation on his tongue and around his mouth as if his tongue had been scalded. Over a similar period his walking had progressively deteriorated and he had become unsteady, tending to trip over; he had sprained his ankles. He knew that his grip was weakening and that muscles in his legs and hands were wasting. There were no other neurological symptoms except frequency of micturition and an aching pain in the low back. There was no disturbance of bowel function and although he had lost a little weight, his appetite had remained reasonable. At the age of 50 years he had had pulmonary tuberculosis treated with INH and PAS. His recent urinary frequency had been attributed to infection, as on one occasion proteinuria had been noticed and he had been given two courses of nalidixic acid. No organisms had been identified on urine culture. He had smoked 20 cigarettes a day for most of his life and drank 2 pints of beer each evening, with an occasional whisky. He had been a clerk in the Civil Service and had neither travelled outside the United Kingdom nor been exposed to any known toxic agents.

On examination he was thin. There was an ill-defined mass in the left hypogastrium and some tenderness over the lumbar spine. The cranial nerves were normal. There was wasting of the small muscles of the hands and the muscles of the anterior tibial compartment with distal weakness in all four limbs. Tendon stretch reflexes were absent and plantar reflexes flexor. There was glove and stocking sensory loss over the hands and feet. He sweated normally and there was no postural hypotension.

Questions

1. The following concerning this patient may be true or false:

   (a) The signs suggest mononeuritis multiplex.
   (b) The history suggests the Guillain–Barré syndrome.
   (c) He has a chronic sensorimotor peripheral neuropathy.
   (d) The previous tuberculosis is not significant.
   (e) Urinary frequency is due to prostatism.

Answers

1. (a) **False**
   (b) **True**
   (c) **True**
   (d) **True**
   (e) **False**

This patient has a progressive mixed neuropathy with the unusual feature of sensory symptoms involving the face, one cause of which includes the Guillain–Barré syndrome, although the length of the history would be against this diagnosis. There is an extensive aetiology for this type of neuropathy, including drugs used to treat tuberculosis (used years previously) and metabolic diseases. The latter is suggested by polyuria and frequency: possible causes include diabetes mellitus and hypercalcaemia (paraneoplastic neuropathy). Certain renal abnormalities may also be associated with a neuropathy including chronic renal failure or renal disease associated with paraproteinaemia or vasculitis.

Investigations should be performed to confirm the type of peripheral neuropathy and to determine its cause. Abnormal investigations included ESR 95 mm/h and urea 8.5 mmol/l.

Questions

2. The following concerning the investigations may be true or false:

   (a) Chest radiography should be performed.
   (b) The absence of albumin, glucose, organisms or cells in the urine would exclude renal disease.
   (c) The following neurophysiological findings suggest a demyelinating neuropathy:

       (i) Motor nerve conduction velocities: 48 m/s.
       (ii) Reduced motor nerve action potential amplitude.
       (iii) Active denervation in peripheral muscles.
       (iv) Absent sural sensory nerve action potentials (SNAP) and reduced ulnar and median nerve SNAP amplitude.

   (d) Normal fasting blood glucose excludes a diabetic neuropathy.

Answers

2. (a) **True**
   (b) **False**
   (c) **False**
   (d) **True**

Chest radiography is indicated in patients with a peripheral neuropathy. A history of tuberculosis was a further indication. A significant proportion of patients with a chronic peripheral sensorimotor neuropathy, particularly with involvement of the face, have a paraneoplastic syndrome; half of these have a lung tumour. The absence of albuminuria is not sufficient to exclude a paraproteinaemia. Electrophysiological studies indicate an axonal neuropathy with normal nerve conduction velocity, absent or reduced SNAP amplitude and evidence of denervation. A normal fasting sugar excludes diabetes.

Bence-Jones proteins were present in the urine, and the serum contained a monoclonal band of kappa chains. There was a dense lesion in the body of L2. Abdominal ultrasound showed that the mass in the left hypochondrium was an enlarged spleen. A diagnosis of myeloma was made; after treatment with chemotherapy the neuropathy improved slightly.

Comment

Paraneoplastic and toxic neuropathies, e.g. those attributable to alcohol and drugs, are usually axonal, whereas those caused by metabolic disease, e.g. diabetes, or those which are postinfective, tend to be demyelinating.

Further reading

SCHAUMBERG, H. H., SPENCER, P. S. and THOMAS, P. K., 'Neuropathies associated with malignancy and dysproteinaemia', *Disorders of Peripheral Nerves* (1983), F. A. Davies Co., Philadelphia, Chapter 13

Exercise 12

Case 12.1 Sudden collapse

A 45-year-old motor mechanic was admitted as an emergency, having collapsed while at work. He was bending over a car, replacing a spark plug, when he suddenly developed a severe occipital headache and dropped the spanner he was holding. He walked a few steps, sat down and then vomited without warning. By the time his workmate had reached him he had slumped to the floor unconscious. An ambulance was called and he was brought to the Accident and Emergency Department where his level of consciousness was found to have improved. He was able to give his name and to describe a severe occipital headache. The left eyelid drooped and the left pupil was dilated and reacted to light neither directly nor consensually. Neurological examination was otherwise normal. There was marked neck stiffness. Blood pressure was 160/110 mmHg.

Questions

1. The following statements may be true or false:
    (a) The eye signs suggest a partial IIIrd nerve palsy.
    (b) Neck stiffness suggests meningeal irritation.
    (c) The investigation of choice is a lumbar puncture.
    (d) Cranial CT is required to exclude an intracerebral haematoma.
    (e) Carotid angiography is indicated.

Answers

1. (a) **True**
   (b) **True**
   (c) **False**
   (d) **True**
   (e) **True**

The patient has suffered a subarachnoid haemorrhage. The signs indicate a partial IIIrd nerve palsy which is strongly suggestive of a ruptured posterior communicating artery aneurysm compressing the IIIrd nerve over which it passes. Patients who have suffered a subarachnoid haemorrhage require no emergency treatment, merely analgesics and anti-emetics. Patients who deteriorate usually do so as a result of arterial spasm and cerebral infarction. CT should be performed to demonstrate subarachnoid blood and hydrocephalus or a haematoma. If blood is demonstrated by CT, lumbar puncture is unnecessary, but if the former is not available lumbar puncture should be performed. It should be undertaken only when sufficient time has elapsed to allow intracranial blood to reach the lumbar subarachnoid space. Timing of angiography is controversial. Most neurosurgeons now perform this within a few days of the initial haemorrhage. In patients who are alert and awake, surgical treatment is indicated at an early stage. Patients with severe neurological deficit including coma do not require early investigation other than CT to exclude hydrocephalus.

Comment

For patients without a major neurological deficit after subarachnoid haemorrhage, the mortality rate for surgical treatment of intracranial aneurysms is now 1–2%; this is therefore the treatment of choice.

Further reading

MOHR, P. J., KISTLER, J. P., ZABRANSKI, J. M., SPETZLER, R. F. and BARNETT, H. J. M., 'Subarachnoid haemorrhage' (eds Barnett, H. J. M., Mohr, J. P., Stein, B. M. and Yatsu, F. M.) Stroke, Pathophysiology, Diagnosis and Management, (1986), Churchill Livingstone, Edinburgh, 656

Case 12.2 Pain in the face

A 53-year-old man previously in good health developed pain in and around his left eye. He had a small pupil with enophthalmos and ptosis but sweating was normal on the left side of his face. There were no other signs.

Questions

1. What is the site of the lesion?
2. What are the probable diagnoses?
3. What investigations should be performed?

Answers

1. He has involvement of the sympathetic nerve supply to the eye. Sympathetic fibres leave the intermediolateral column of the spinal grey matter via the ventral nerve roots and the white rami communicantes at T1 and run via the three cervical ganglia into the carotid sheath at the base of the skull where they become the internal carotid nerves. Fibres to the sweat glands leave at this point. Fibres to the eye run with the ophthalmic artery to the tarsal muscles and either with the nasociliary nerve or through the ciliary ganglion to the dilator pupillae and the vessels of the eyeball.
2. (a) An infraclinoid aneurysm of the internal carotid artery, a fusiform dilation of the artery itself, rather than a saccular aneurysm.
   (b) Raeder's syndrome (paratrigeminal neuralgia), when no underlying cause is found.
3. Carotid angiography.

Comment

It is rare to find an underlying aneurysm and most patients require treatment with analgesics only.

Further reading

VIJAYAN, N. and WATSON, C. 'Raeder's syndrome, pericarotid syndromes and carotidynia' (eds Vinken, P. J., Bruyn, G. W., Klawans, H. L. and Rose, F. C.), *Handbook of Neurology, Vol. 4(48)* (1986), Elsevier Science Pubs, Amsterdam, Chapter 21

Case 12.3 An incontinent child

A 12-year-old girl was brought to the Paediatric Out-Patient
Department by her parents because of incontinence. She stopped
being enuretic at the age of 3 years but became incontinent again
at the age of 5 years. Her bladder control was otherwise
completely normal. There was no incontinence to strain, cough or
sneezing. If she began to laugh involuntarily, however, her bladder
emptied completely and she was unable to control this. There
were no other symptoms. She was a perfectly healthy child and
physical examination was normal.

Questions

1. What is the diagnosis?
2. What investigations should be performed?
3. What is the prognosis?
4. What treatment should be given?

232

Answers

1. This is giggle micturition and often has a family history. The cause is unknown although it has been likened to 'cataplexy' of the bladder.
2. In typical cases no investigations are required.
3. The prognosis is variable although it usually ceases in adult life.
4. No particular treatments are helpful.

Comment

It is a rare condition but should be considered when a child presents with diurnal incontinence.

Further reading

McKEITH, R. C., 'Micturition induced by giggling', *Guy's Hospital Report* (1964), **113**, 250–252

Case 12.4 An unsteady lady

A 62-year-old lady was brought to the surgery by her daughter because of increasing unsteadiness. She had always been overweight and in the previous 6 months her weight had increased and, more importantly to her family, her mobility had been grossly impaired by unsteadiness which had increased over the preceding 6–8 weeks. Initially she had been unwilling to leave home by herself and latterly reluctant to get up from her bed, and she was unable to descend the stairs unaided. Although she was unsteady walking short distances, she strongly denied any dizziness. Her family and friends felt that her speech was slurred and she complained of headaches. There was no significant past medical history other than a cholecystectomy 25 years previously, and 5 years previously she had been treated for thyrotoxicosis. She drank a bottle of Guinness each night. She did not smoke.

She was sallow with thin grey hair and plump cold hands. Pulse was 56/min and in sinus rhythm. Auscultation of the heart and great vessels was normal. Blood pressure was 179/70 mmHg; peripheral pulses were palpable. She was ataxic in all four limbs and had a slurring dysarthria but no nystagmus. Reflexes were slow in relaxing and her voice, when she could be persuaded to talk, was hoarse. The soft palate elevated centrally.

Questions

1. The following statements concerning this patient may be true or false:

   (a) She has a subacute cerebellar syndrome.
   (b) The cause of her symptoms is alcohol abuse.
   (c) The absence of a family history would exclude a degenerative ataxia.
   (d) Weight gain, hoarseness and slow relaxing reflexes suggest a metabolic cause.
   (e) A history of epilepsy would be of relevance.

Answers

1. (a) **True**
   (b) **False**
   (c) **False**
   (d) **True**
   (e) **True**

A progressive ataxia involving gait, limbs and speech, without nystagmus or signs of raised intracranial pressure, suggests a subacute cerebellar degeneration. This may occur on a familial or degenerative basis or be attributable to toxic or metabolic causes. Hereditary ataxias may be recessively inherited: thus the absence of a family history does not exclude this. The history may be unreliable but it does not support alcohol abuse and there is no other evidence of this, e.g. peripheral neuropathy or eye-movement disorder. Phenytoin and hypothyroidism (the latter suggested by weight gain, a hoarse voice and slow relaxing reflexes) are also rare causes of a subacute cerebellar degeneration.

Investigation revealed serum thyroxine 20 nmol/l and TSH >20 u/l; cranial CT showed mild cerebral and cerebellar atrophy; CSF was normal; chest radiography was normal; ESR, 36 mm/h; serum B_{12} normal; there was no evidence of underlying neoplasia.

Comment

An inherited ataxia cannot be excluded but myxoedema is a recognized cause of a subacute cerebellar syndrome. A para-neoplastic syndrome should also be considered, as signs may develop many years before the tumour becomes apparent.

Further reading

GILMAN, S., BLOEDEL, J. R. and LECHTENBERG, R., 'Metabolic disorders', *Disorders of the Cerebellum* (1981), F. A. Davies Co., Philadelphia, Chapter 16

Case 12.5 Difficulty in swallowing

A 62-year-old right-handed labourer was referred to hospital as an emergency with the diagnosis of a brain-stem stroke. A few weeks previously he had developed difficulty in swallowing and speaking; had become aware of double vision whilst watching television in the evening, and then had increasing difficulty in chewing his food. He tended to slur his speech and dribble saliva while talking. The illness had gradually progressed to such an extent that the double vision was present most of the day and his speech was difficult to understand. On the day of admission he choked while eating lunch. He had no symptoms in his arms or legs. There was no headache or sensory loss. He had previously suffered from arthritis and had been treated with a variety of different medications for this. During the 6 months before referral he had been requiring increased medication. His sister and mother both had thyroid disease.

Questions

1. The following concerning the history may be true or false:
   - (a) The progression of the symptoms would be compatible with a brain-stem infarct.
   - (b) The lack of history of fatigue or generalized weakness would make the diagnosis of myasthenia gravis unlikely.
   - (c) The history suggests a pseudobulbar palsy.
   - (d) Medication for arthritis is unlikely to be relevant to his presenting symptoms.
   - (e) A family history of thyroid disease may be relevant.

Answers

1. (a) **False**
   (b) **False**
   (c) **False**
   (d) **False**
   (e) **True**

Varying eye movement symptoms should always suggest myasthenia, regardless of the absence of a history of fatigue. Patients on penicillamine for arthritis may develop myasthenia, and a family history of thyroid disease is not uncommon. The history is too long, and symptoms too anatomically discrete, for a brain-stem stroke. In a pseudobulbar palsy there is incontinence of emotion and affect, and spasticity in the limbs in addition to bulbar signs.

General examination was normal. There were no signs of hypo- or hyperthyroidism. There was a fatiguing weakness of the facial muscles and ptosis and paralytic diplopia after exercise. He was dysphagic and had a flaccid dysarthria which became worse during speech. Power in the limbs was normal. Tendon stretch reflexes were normal.

Questions

2. Concerning the diagnosis, the following statements may be true or false:

   (a) Normal reflexes make a diagnosis of the Eaton–Lambert syndrome unlikely.
   (b) A diagnosis of myasthenia gravis may be made by demonstrating the presence of acetylcholine receptor antibodies in the serum.
   (c) Administration of intravenous edrophonium is indicated.
   (d) Tetanic train stimulation may show an incremental response.
   (e) Thoracic CT would be expected to show a thymic hyperplasia.

Answers

2. (a) **True**
   (b) **True**
   (c) **True**
   (d) **False**
   (e) **False**

The presumptive diagnosis is that of myasthenia gravis. In the Eaton–Lambert (myasthenic) syndrome reflexes are absent but appear on testing after exercise. The diagnosis may be confirmed by the response to administration of intravenous edrophonium (1 mg test dose followed by 5–10 mg after 30 s), or by finding antibodies to the acetylcholine receptor. Neurophysiological abnormalities include a decremental response to tetanic train stimulation at 5–10 Hz, and evidence of neuromuscular blockade is seen on single-fibre EMG in the form of jitter and blocking of motor action potentials. Thoracic CT is indicated in all patients with myasthenia. Thymic hyperplasia would be expected in a younger patient; a thymoma can occur at any age.

Comment

Myasthenia may cause any form of eye movement disorder or bulbar weakness. Symptomatic treatment includes an anti-cholinesterase, e.g. pyridostigmine, given up to five times daily. Definitive treatment includes immunosuppression with steroids and azathioprine. Older patients respond less well to thymectomy.

Further reading

BROWN, J. C. and WYNN-PARRY, C. B., 'Neuromuscular stimulation and transmission' (ed. Walton, J. N.), *Disorders of Voluntary Muscle* (1981), Churchill Livingstone, Edinburgh, Chapter 26

Case 12.6 Intermittent weakness of the left arm

A 56-year-old butcher came to the clinic with the complaint of intermittent weakness of the left arm. Six weeks earlier he had been working in his shop when his left arm became weak and he dropped a tray of sausages. He also became aware of a slight weakness of the left leg and had to sit down. Within a few minutes his symptoms had started to improve and within 5 min he had made a complete recovery. On the way home he had a further attack in the car while driving; he was unable to steer and his left foot slipped off the clutch. He managed to stop the car and symptoms again settled within a few minutes. He called for help and a passer-by took him to his general practitioner. No abnormal signs were noted and he was referred to a neurology clinic. Further attacks occurred in the week before his appointment and in the last attack he had blurring of vision in the right eye.

On examination he appeared healthy. Blood pressure was 130/85 mmHg. There was no cardiac abnormality. There was a short bruit in the left supraclavicular fossa and a long systolic bruit behind the angle of the right jaw. A similar bruit was heard over the right orbit.

Questions

1. What are these attacks?
2. What is the relationship between the weakness in the left arm and the blurring of vision in the right eye?
3. What is the significance of the bruit at the angle of the right jaw?
4. What is the prognosis?
5. What should be the management?

240

Answers

1. The attacks of weakness are transient cerebral ischaemia probably in the distribution of the right internal carotid artery.
2. The attack in which weakness of the left arm was accompanied by blurring of vision in the right eye, suggests concurrent ischaemia affecting the right central retinal artery, a branch of the right internal carotid artery.
3. The bruit suggests carotid artery stenosis, and is probably merely transmitted to the orbit, although it may indicate intracranial stenosis.
4. The prognosis for patients with transient ischaemic attacks is variable but current epidemiological studies would suggest an incidence of stroke of between 3% and 5% per year. There is no evidence to suggest that this prognosis is worse in patients with carotid artery stenosis. There is also a risk of sudden death due to a cardiac arrhythmia or myocardial ischaemia.
5. The management of these patients is controversial. Readily treatable risk factors include anaemia, polycythaemia, diabetes mellitus and hypertension. Aspirin may reduce the risk of stroke and sudden death and is a relatively safe form of treatment.

Comment

Carotid angiography showed carotid stenosis. The role of carotid endarterectomy in these patients has not been proved. The European Carotid Artery Surgery Trial is currently evaluating the risks and benefits of this form of treatment, and it would not be unreasonable to treat patients medically until the results of this trial are available.

Further reading

BARNETT, H. J. M., 'Antithrombotic therapy in cerebral vascular disease. Antispasmodics and fibrinolytics', (eds Barnett, H. J. M., Mohr, J. P., Stein, B. M. and Yatsu, F. M.), *Stroke, Pathophysiology, Diagnosis and Management* (1986), Churchill Livingstone, Edinburgh, Chapter 50.

Index by subject

Numbers in **bold** type indicate main diagnosis or major discussion of topic

241